T0369419

Register Now for Online Access to Your Book!

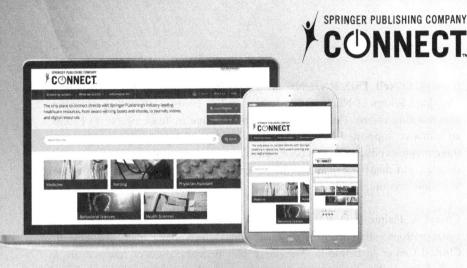

SPRINGER PUBLISHING COMPANY
CONNECT™

Your print purchase of *Developing Online Courses in Nursing Education, Fourth Edition* **includes online access to the contents of your book**—increasing accessibility, portability, and searchability!

Access today at:

http://connect.springerpub.com/content/book/978-0-8261-4057-9
or scan the QR code at the right with your smartphone
and enter the access code below.

Scan here for quick access.

04NJ2LM8

SPRINGER PUBLISHING COMPANY
View all our products at springerpub.com

Carol A. O'Neil, PhD, RN, CNE, is an associate professor at the University of Maryland School of Nursing. She teaches online courses in nursing education and teaching online. Dr. O'Neil is a Web Initiative in Teaching (WIT) Fellow, an initiative supported by the University System of Maryland. In addition to three previous editions of this book, she has to her credit a journal article, a book chapter, and many national and international presentations related to teaching in online environments.

Cheryl A. Fisher, EdD, RN-BC, is the senior nurse consultant for extramural collaborations within the nursing department at the National Institutes of Health Clinical Center in Bethesda, Maryland. Her primary areas of research are in course development, program evaluation, and administrative areas of clinical research nursing. Prior to her current position, Dr. Fisher worked as the program director for professional development, working to enhance educational opportunities through the use of technology. She received her doctorate in instructional technology from Towson University and has a postgraduate certificate in nursing informatics from the University of Maryland and a postgraduate certificate in nursing education from George Mason University. She is responsible for outreach to the extramural National Institutes of Health sites and internationally to provide education and resources for nurses.

Matthew J. Rietschel, MS, is the assistant dean, information and learning technology, and an assistant professor at the University of Maryland School of Nursing. He received his bachelor's degree in education from Salisbury University and his master's degree in instructional technology from Towson University, where he is currently working on his doctorate in instructional technology. He currently supervises the development and deployment of all web-based and blended courses, manages the information technology infrastructure, supports a multitude of grant projects involving technology, and teaches in the Teaching in Nursing and Health Professions Certificate program.

Developing Online Courses in Nursing Education

Fourth Edition

Carol A. O'Neil, PhD, RN, CNE

Cheryl A. Fisher, EdD, RN-BC

Matthew J. Rietschel, MS

SPRINGER PUBLISHING COMPANY

Springer Publishing Company, LLC
11 West 42nd Street
New York, NY 10036
www.springerpub.com
http://connect.springerpub.com

Acquisitions Editor: Joe Morita
Compositor: Amnet Systems

ISBN: 978-0-8261-4039-5
ebook ISBN: 978-0-8261-4057-9
Instructor's Manual ISBN: 978-0-8261-4038-8
DOI: 10.1891/9780826140579

Instructor's Materials: Qualified instructors may request supplements by emailing textbook@springerpub.com

19 20 21 22 / 5 4 3 2 1

The author and the publisher of this Work have made every effort to use sources believed to be reliable to provide information that is accurate and compatible with the standards generally accepted at the time of publication. Because medical science is continually advancing, our knowledge base continues to expand. Therefore, as new information becomes available, changes in procedures become necessary. We recommend that the reader always consult current research and specific institutional policies before performing any clinical procedure. The author and publisher shall not be liable for any special, consequential, or exemplary damages resulting, in whole or in part, from the readers' use of, or reliance on, the information contained in this book. The publisher has no responsibility for the persistence or accuracy of URLs for external or third-party Internet websites referred to in this publication and does not guarantee that any content on such websites is, or will remain, accurate or appropriate.

Library of Congress Cataloging-in-Publication Data
Names: O'Neil, Carol A., author. | Fisher, Cheryl A., author. | Rietschel, Matthew J., author.
Title: Developing online courses in nursing education / Carol A. O'Neil, Cheryl A. Fisher, Matthew J. Rietschel.
Other titles: Developing online learning environments in nursing education
Description: Fourth edition. | New York, NY : Springer Publishing Company, [2020] | Preceded by Developing online learning environments in nursing education / Carol A. O'Neil, Cheryl A. Fisher, Matthew J. Rietschel. 3rd ed. c2014. | Includes bibliographical references.
Identifiers: LCCN 2019010558 (print) | LCCN 2019011511 (ebook) | ISBN 9780826140579 (eBook) | ISBN 9780826140395 (print : alk. paper) | ISBN 9780826140579 (e-book) | ISBN 9780826140388 (instructor's manual)
Subjects: | MESH: Education, Nursing—methods | Internet | Education, Distance—methods | Curriculum
Classification: LCC RT73 (ebook) | LCC RT73 (print) | NLM WY 18 | DDC 610.73071/1—dc23
LC record available at https://lccn.loc.gov/2019010558

Contact us to receive discount rates on bulk purchases.
We can also customize our books to meet your needs.
For more information please contact: sales@springerpub.com

Printed in the United States of America.

*We dedicate this book to our
spouses, children, and grandchildren,
who have supported us to persevere with our
commitment to online education.*

Contents

Contributors

Susan L. Bindon, DNP, RN-BC, is an assistant professor at the University of Maryland School of Nursing, teaching online graduate courses in nursing education. She has 20 years of nursing education experience in academic and staff development settings and in classroom, clinical, and online learning environments. She was director of education at a Baltimore-area health system, where she was responsible for the competency and continuing education of the clinical staff and had oversight for the organization's learning management system. Dr. Bindon is active in the Association for Nursing Professional Development and is currently serving a 2-year term on the board of directors. She has served 5 years on the editorial board for the *Journal for Nurses in Staff Development (JNSD)* and acted as JNSD's website editor, as well. Dr. Bindon is American Nurses Credentialing Center (ANCC) certified in nursing professional development and is a review course instructor for ANCC's Nursing Professional Development Certification exam.

Kathleen M. Buckley, PhD, RN, is an associate professor in the School of Nursing at the University of Maryland, where she has been a key player in developing and teaching blended courses in the Doctor of Nursing Practice program. She has expertise in the use of web conferencing and active learning strategies in online and blended courses. Dr. Buckley is also certified as a reviewer for Quality Matters, a leader in quality assurance for online education, and has participated as an external reviewer for a number of online and blended nursing courses throughout the United States.

Kathleen A. Gould, EdD, MA, RD, LDN, is a clinical associate professor in the Department of Health Sciences at Towson University. Dr. Gould is a registered dietitian and teaches nutrition to prenursing and other health professional students. She is also responsible for coordinating and supervising community health students in their internship experiences. Dr. Gould has experience teaching online and implementing problem-based learning in this environment. Her research is focused on student self-directed learning readiness, success in online problem-based learning, and interprofessional education.

William A. Sadera, PhD, is professor of instructional technology at Towson University. Dr. Sadera also serves as the director of the doctoral program in instructional technology in Towson University's College of Education. Dr. Sadera has been active in the field of instructional technology and online learning, having taught courses, conducted research projects, and published on these topics for 20 years; his current research focuses on online professional development, pedagogy, and effective design of online instruction.

Shannon Tucker, MS, CPHIMS, is the assistant dean of instructional design and technology and an affiliate assistant professor at the University of Maryland School of Pharmacy, where she supervises educational technology integration and academic application development; supports academic operations, including new program development; and teaches coursework in professional communication. She earned a master's degree in interface design and information architecture from the University of Baltimore and a bachelor's degree in visual arts from the University of Maryland Baltimore County. Her current doctoral work in instructional technology at Towson University synthesizes her expertise in user experience design with instructional design to create engaging learning environments.

Preface

A comment in the preface of the last edition was that some things are the same and some things are different. In this edition, the conclusion is that some things are the same, and they are the basics of teaching and learning online. However, some things are not only different, they are very different in relation to technology, students, and structure of online learning environments. Some things that are the same are areas of reconceptualization, pedagogy, interaction, course management, assessment of students, and evaluation of courses. In these areas, a review of the literature revealed the most updated best practices, and they are included in this current edition.

The very different things include technology and new structures for teaching and learning. Emphasis on demographics of online learners, expectations of employers, automation, technology, and a focus on lifelong learning is leading to changes in what and how we teach. Institutions of higher learning can no longer teach all the knowledge and skills needed to meet the demands of the employer. Thus, there is a need for lifelong learning and flexible and creative learning environments.

What is on the horizon? In addition to traditional education, massive online open courses (MOOCs), certificates, badges, and stackable degrees will provide education for the purpose of training and retraining. If completed, the new knowledge and skills can be transformed into continuing education or degree programs.

This edition is still about using the web and all its richness to teach students and professional nurses how to use technology and to maintain competency and embrace lifelong learning as a nursing professional. Definitions, history, and best practices for teaching online are described, and they form a foundational knowledge base for teaching (Chapter 1, Introduction to Teaching and Learning in Online Environments). The impacts of demographics, finance, technology, and career development on teaching and learning using alternative teaching structures are identified (Chapter 2, The Impact of New Directions on Teaching and Learning). Pedagogy and the study of learning provides the theory to develop effective educational programs (Chapter 3, Reflections on Pedagogy in Online Instruction). Theories and frameworks that guide the development and use of flexible learning environments are introduced (Chapter 4, Flexible Learning Environments). Guiding structures of online learning, such as interaction and feedback, are applicable when developing traditional and alternative learning environments (Chapter 5, Guiding Structures for New Learning Environments).

Other chapters deal with reconceptualizing course content from face-to-face to an online environment (Chapter 6, Reconceptualizing the Online Learning Environment); creating blended-learning environments (Chapter 7, Practical Applications in Academic Online Learning Environments); developing, teaching, and evaluating professional education (Chapter 8, Practical Applications in Professional Online Learning Environments); and establishing the pedagogical foundations of teaching continuing medical education (Chapter 9, Theoretical Applications of Continuing Education). The technology courseware and software necessary to teach in online environments (Chapter 10, Technical Considerations to Support Learning Environments), manage online learning (Chapter 11, Course Management Methods), and assess and evaluate learning in online environments (Chapter 12, Assessment and Evaluation of Online Learning) are pertinent topics for teaching online. The last chapter (Chapter 13, The Changing Role of the Nurse Educator) introduces the characteristics that the nurse educator needs in developing and teaching in flexible and creative environments and explains how nurse educators are supporting the direction of the future trends for nursing.

We hope you enjoy the practicality of this book and have fun in the process!

Carol A. O'Neil
Cheryl A. Fisher
Matthew J. Rietschel

Qualified instructors may obtain access to supplementary material (Instructor's Manual) by emailing textbook@springerpub.com.

Introduction to Teaching and Learning in Online Environments

Carol A. O'Neil

INTRODUCTION

This chapter explores the basic concepts and the current landscape of teaching and learning in online environments.

DEFINITION OF TERMS

Distance education is the delivery of content using technology (Seaman, Allen, & Seaman, 2018). Learning takes place when the learner and the teacher are geographically separated (Layton, 2017). The Sloan Consortium (Allen & Seaman, 2018) defines online learning in terms of the proportion of content delivered online. When 80% or more of the content is online, it is an online course. When 30% to 79% is online, the course is hybrid or blended. When 1% to 29% of the content is online, the course is web facilitated, and when no part of the course is online, it is a traditional class. Web-based learning means using the World Wide Web as the teaching and learning strategy. There is a reduction in time and space barriers to learning, and learning can take place anytime and anywhere.

HISTORICAL PERSPECTIVE OF TEACHING WITH TECHNOLOGY

The practice of teaching and learning at a distance is not new to education. Paper-based distance curricula in which the learner enrolled in a university and received learning packages in the mail have been available for some time. Early correspondence courses included interaction with the instructor through telephone calls and mail. Television also provided a medium for teaching and learning at a distance. Students in remote areas could use the television to obtain learning content. In the late 1960s, Schramm (1962) conducted studies that compared instructional television (ITV) with classroom instruction and summarized the results of more than 400 empirical studies. The findings of his research revealed no significant difference between learning from a television or in a classroom.

As distance education progressed from correspondence courses to online learning, opportunities for interpersonal interaction also increased. Videoconferencing made it possible for learners and faculty members to interact in real time. With the emergence of the Internet, particularly email and the World Wide Web, it became possible to promote high degrees of interaction using mainstream technology and cost-effective learning environments.

Following Schramm's (1962) conclusions that there was no significant difference in learning between the traditional classroom and televised learning, researchers compared classroom instruction to other methods of distance education. Numerous studies comparing traditional classroom-based instruction with technology-supported instruction have found no significant difference in critical educational variables, such as learning outcomes. Wetzel, Radtke, and Stern (1994) summarized the results of comparative studies conducted through the mid-1990s and found no significant differences in learning outcomes between the two learning environments. Thomas Russell (1998) at North Carolina State University studied hundreds of sources of written material about distance education and concluded that the learning outcomes of students in the traditional classroom are similar to those of students in distance technology classes. This was termed the *no-significant-differences phenomenon*.

The American Federation of Teachers and the National Education Association commissioned the Institute of Higher Education Policy to conduct a review of the current research on the effectiveness of distance education (Merisotis & Phipps, 1999). Merisotis and Phipps (1999) reviewed studies published in the 1990s and presented "What's the Difference: A Review of Contemporary Research on the Effectiveness of Distance Learning in Education." The findings were that online students tend to perform as effectively as traditional students. Online students had similar learning experiences and were as satisfied with their learning experiences as were traditional classroom learners. The authors noted several shortcomings in the original research: lack of control for extraneous variables, lack of randomization of subjects, questionable validity and reliability of instruments used to measure student outcome and attitude, and no control for reactive effects, such as the impact of motivation and interest, because taking a course online is a novelty. The authors suggest that because of these shortcomings, the study was inconclusive. The question—what is the best way to teach students—prevailed (Merisotis & Phipps, 1999).

This led to the investigation of other variables, such as overall course satisfaction, course organization, and attainment of class objectives. Leasure, Davis, and Thievon (2000) looked at these variables in traditional lecture and distance-based instruction and reported no significant differences. Allen, Bourhis, Burrell, and Mabry (2002) conducted a meta-analysis and found no differences in satisfaction levels but found a slight preference for traditional face-to-face courses over distance-based education courses.

Researchers began to move beyond comparative studies and into other methods, such as discourse analysis and in-depth interviews. These methods have provided theoretical frameworks for practice. Billings (2000) suggested a model that focuses on the best practices that included technology, faculty, students, and outcomes. The author developed examples of evidence for the best practices in the model. For example, evidence for the technology best practice is infrastructure that includes access to the Internet, course management software, user support, and appropriate hardware and software.

While the guiding principles of quality practice were under development, universities were struggling with what Noble (1998) calls automation. According to Noble, "automation—the distribution of digitized course material online, without the participation of professors who develop such material—is often justified as an inevitable part of the new 'knowledge-based' society" (Noble, 1998, p. 1). The University of California at Los Angeles (UCLA) instituted the Instructional Enhancement Initiative, which mandated that all arts and sciences courses have a web-based delivery component. The university collaborated with private corporations and formed its own for-profit company (Noble, 1998). Noble says, "It is by no accident that the high-tech transformation of higher education is being initiated and implemented from the top down, either without any student and faculty involvement in the decision-making or despite it" (Noble, 1998, p. 2). Although faculty members and students were opposed to the initiative, UCLA administrators continued with their plans (Noble, 1998). Further, Noble cites a reason for the decision to continue—the fear of being left behind in an academic trend he calls "the commercialism of higher education" (Noble, 1998). The function of the university is to teach, and universities are developing their course-ware into marketable, sellable products in hopes of getting "a piece of the commercial action for their institutions or themselves, as vendors in their own right of software and content" (Noble, 1998, p. 5). The concern of faculty members is the quality of education. They view web-based instruction as commoditizing education, and the fear was that the quality of instruction will be compromised by automation.

Online courses and programs grew from 1999 to 2001 through grants awarded by the Department of Education called Learning Anytime Anywhere Partnerships (LAAP) for innovative distance learning projects that included partnerships. With funding from President Bill Clinton's Fund for the Improvement of Postsecondary Education, LAAP received $10 million in 1999, $23.3 million in 2000, and $30 million in 2001. Even with the phasing out of the program, the emphasis on partnerships in projects continued to grow (Carnevale, 2001).

What Is an Online Course?

The original purpose of the web was to communicate and share information. The development of the web dramatically changed the methods of communication and sharing information and ultimately changed the practice of education. Online learning is instructor moderated, instructor taught, and instructor mentored, yet student self-directed. An online learning environment can comprise large discussion groups, small group discussions, individual activities, group activities, and various levels of interaction between and among students, faculty, and the content. Content dissemination includes a variety of strategies, including video casting, audiotaping, films, and links to the web, charts, graphs, statistical data, formulas, and case studies. Interaction can be synchronous (real time) or asynchronous (delayed). Synchronous interaction means having a live discussion online, where the faculty facilitator and students can hear and/or see each other in real time. Asynchronous communication entails leaving messages at specific posting sites that others in the learning environment can read at their convenience, such as discussion boards, blogs, and wikis.

Online learning environments comprise individual courses, groups of courses, and entire programs. The degree of Internet use in a course ranges from supplementing classroom learning to courses/programs that are completely online. Online learners can attend traditional universities, such as Pennsylvania State University (www.worldcampus.psu.edu), or virtual universities, such as California Virtual University (www.cvc.edu). In addition to online courses and programs, online journals are available that focus on teaching and learning online, such as the *Online Learning Journal*. There are professional organizations that provide resources for online teaching and learning, such as EDUCAUSE (www.educause.edu) and the Online Learning Consortium (onlinelearningconsortium.org). Some courses can be taken online free of charge at websites such as Coursera (www.coursera.org).

Why Take a Course Online?

There are several reasons for taking a course online. One is that our students are digital natives. They grew up using smartphones, laptops, and tablets and viewing YouTube videos and playing games. Social media is an integral part of their communication and interactions. Online learning is an extension of day-to-day activities to learning activities. The second is the flexibility and pace of learning in online environments. Students can work, have families, continue with their home lives, and be able to learn anytime and anywhere. The third reason is the impact of technology on learning. Online learning environments allow for the use of technology to enhance learning that is creative with the ability to include learning strategies to meet differing learning styles.

There are both advantages and disadvantages to online learning. The advantages are:

- Accessible 24 hours a day and 7 days a week
- Accessible anywhere with Internet access
- Learning is student centered
- Access to resources and links on the Internet
- Opportunities for high-quality interactive dialogue

The disadvantages are:

- Need to be computer literate
- System failures

- Need hardware and software
- Learning style of student may not match online learning

Who Is Learning Online?

Student enrollment in distance learning classes has increased for the 14th year. This accounts for 15% of students taking only online courses and 17% of students taking some courses online. A recent meta-analysis by the U.S. Department of Education found that students perform better in online learning environments. A key contributor to success is the flexibility of learning online. The student can determine the time and place to learn (Seaman et al., 2018). Students think that online learning is as good as or better than traditional classroom learning (Schaffhauser, 2018).

Where Are Learners Learning?

Students are learning in fully online programs in which they take all the courses in the program online, in programs in which they take some courses online and some courses in traditional classrooms, and in blended courses in which some of the course is online and some is in a face-to-face setting.

Learning online also takes place in environments that are nontraditional. The foundational theory of education and the processes of teaching are the same in these settings as in traditional environments. What changes is the structure of the learning environment. A need for a change in structure stems in part from the cost of education and employment opportunities. About 60% of employment positions require education beyond high school (Young, 2018). Tuition is rising, and this cost can be a barrier to enrolling and graduating from a degree program. These have led to alternative structures in education. One is competency-based learning, which focuses on the mastery of academic and performance skills. Learning is personalized and individualized and self-paced and is evaluated through performance. The learner earns recognition or credit by performance that validates mastery. Descriptions of some of the alternative structures follow.

Coursera is an organization that offers quality online courses that are accessible and affordable.

MOOCs are massive open online courses. They are new pathways to higher education. Students register for an online course without enrolling in a university or a program. MOOCs are accessible online and are cost-effective. MOOCs connect learners globally who learn and share in online environments. EdX is yet another platform that offers free courses but charges for certificates (Skiba, 2017).

Badges and microcredentials are indicators of achievement of learning. For example, EDUCAUSE awards badges when a learner completes a program.

Stackable degrees are certificate programs that when completed can be added to other certificates so that a degree program can be developed.

Who Is Teaching Online?

Although students are enrolling in online courses and administrators support online learning, faculty attitude of teaching and learning online has not significantly changed. About 9% of faculty educators surveyed by Inside Higher Ed (Jaschik & Lederman, 2014) strongly agreed that students have an equivalent learning experience online, and 83% responded that online courses are of a lower quality than traditional courses. About 33% responded that they have taught an online class.

How Do Students Learn?

Chickering and Ehrman (1996) used the American Association for Higher Education (AAHE) Principles for Good Practice to develop best practices to teach students in online environments and developed a paper called "Implementing the Seven Principles: Technology as Lever." The following points are the best practices and examples:

1. *Good practice encourages contact between students and faculty.*
   Students and faculty exchange thoughts and ideas more effectively and safely in online environments than in the traditional classroom. Communication becomes more intimate, protected, and connected online than in face-to-face interaction.
2. *Good practice develops reciprocity and cooperation among students.*
   Technology provides opportunities for interaction in online learning environments. Students can share their knowledge and experiences in small groups, in study groups, during group problem-solving exercises, and in activities related to learning content. For example, the learning content may be epidemiology and the epidemiologic triangle: the agent, the host, and the environment. Online students

can complete an assignment on the epidemiology of West Nile virus, describe how the infection occurs, and suggest strategies to prevent it from occurring.

3. *Good practice uses active learning techniques.*

The technology included in online learning systems provides opportunity for active learning. For example, students in an online community health nursing course are given an exercise to assess a community. Student directions include obtaining census and vital statistics data. Students then view a windshield survey video (made by the faculty). The exercise is to use both of these sources of information to formulate a summary of the key points about the community. The group posts the summary in a public discussion forum for all groups to read.

4. *Good practice gives prompt feedback.*

Technology provides many opportunities for feedback, both synchronous (real time) and asynchronous (time delayed) and via email. Defining "prompt" feedback in the course directions or in the syllabus enhances clarity. For example, the instructor might post the following message: "I will read all postings on the discussion board and post a comment to the group at the end of the week," or the faculty might post "I will answer all emails within 3 working days."

5. *Good practice emphasizes time on task.*

Time is critical, and using time wisely is important. Online courses save the students commuting time and parking costs. Students can learn anywhere—at home, at work, or virtually anywhere there is an Internet connection. A rule of thumb to determine the number of hours a week that students will spend on an online course is to double or triple the number of course credits. For example, a student enrolled in a 3-credit course can expect to spend 6 to 9 hours each week working on the course.

6. *Good practice communicates high expectations.*

Some students register for online courses because they think it will be easier than traditional courses. They soon find out that this is a fallacy. Clearly communicate expectations to students. If students are not performing at the expected level, the faculty should contact the student, describe observed behavior, and delineate expected behavior. For example, if the faculty reads a student post with comments like "I agree" or "Great idea," the faculty should contact this student. The message that "I have read your postings and see that in some you clearly express your ideas and use the literature to support your ideas, but in other postings your comments are less substantiated" or

"I read that you have excellent ideas and would like to see you share these more with your peers" is shared.

7. *Good practice respects diverse talents and ways of learning.*
The advantage of online courses is the many resources available to accommodate a variety of learning styles. For example, for the visual learners, use PowerPoint, charts, and graphs. For audio learners, use podcasts. For readers, add notes. Links to YouTube videos and a plethora of websites can add value to the content.

Ten years after Chickering and Ehrman principles, Lewis and Abdul-Hamid (2006) updated the principles based on their quantitative study and suggested the following best practices. They are:

1. Foster interaction.
2. Provide feedback.
3. Facilitate learning.
4. Maintain enthusiasm and organization.

The first three (interaction, feedback, and active learning) remained as best practices over the years. Maintaining enthusiasm and organization is an additional best practice.

SUMMARY

Online learning environments have morphed into academia as acceptable methods for achieving academic goals in flexible and creative learning environments. Students are motivated and independent, and faculty members have changed roles from being the sage-on-the-stage (classroom teaching) to guides-on-the-side (online teaching). When considering the research findings over the past several decades along with societal changes and demand for accessible learning, it becomes evident that learning online is heading in a direction that will drive demand. As new generations grow up learning online, educators will continue to face the challenge of keeping students engaged through active learning and feedback that facilitates the learning process.

REFERENCES

Allen, I. E., & Seaman, J. (2018). *Digital learning compass: Distance education enrollment report 2017*. Retrieved from https://onlinelearningconsortium.org/read/digital -learning-compass-distance-education-enrollment-report-2017

Allen, M., Bourhis, J., Burrell, N., & Mabry, E. (2002). Comparing student satisfaction with distance education to traditional classrooms in higher education: A meta analysis. *American Journal of Distance Education, 16*(2), 83–97. doi:10.1207/S15389286AJDE1602_3

Billings, D. M. (2000). A framework for assessing outcomes and practices in web-based courses in nursing. *Journal of Nursing Education, 39*(2), 60–67. doi:10.3928/0148-4834-20000201-07

Carnevale, D. (2001, September 28). Education department cuts new distance education grants. *The Chronicle of Higher Education.* Retrieved from https://www.chronicle.com/article/Education-Department-Cuts-New/35417

Chickering, A. W., & Ehrmann, S. C. (1996). *Implementing the seven principles: Technology as a lever.* Retrieved from http://www.tltgroup.org/programs/seven

Jaschik, S., & Lederman, D. (Eds.). (2014). *The 2014 Inside Higher Ed Survey of Faculty Attitudes on Technology.* Retrieved from https://www.insidehighered.com/audio/2014/11/18/2014-survey-faculty-attitudes-technology

Layton, S. (2017, August 24). *What's the difference between online learning and distance learning?* Retrieved from https://www.aeseducation.com/blog/2013/09/difference-between-online-learning-and-distance-learning

Leasure, A., Davis, L., & Thievon, S. (2000). Comparison of student outcomes and preferences in a traditional vs. World Wide Web-based baccalaureate nursing research course. *Journal of Nursing Education, 39*(4), 149–154.

Lewis, C., & Abdul-Hamid, H. (2006). Implementing effective online teaching practices: Voices of exemplary faculty. *Innovative Higher Education, 31*(2), 83–98. Retrieved from https://link.springer.com/article/10.1007%2Fs10755-006-9010-z. doi:10.1007/s10755-006-9010-z

Merisotis, J. P., & Phipps, R. A. (1999). *What's the difference? A review of contemporary research on the effectiveness of distance learning in higher education.* Washington, DC: The Institute for Higher Education Policy.

Noble, D. F. (1998). Digital diploma mills: The automation of higher education. *First Monday, 3*, 1–7. Retrieved from https://firstmonday.org/ojs/index.php/fm/article/view/569/490

Russell, T. (1998). *No significant difference: Phenomenon as reported in 248 research reports, summaries, and papers* (4th ed.). Raleigh: North Carolina State University.

Schaffhauser, D. (2018). *Survey: Most students say online learning is as good or better than face-to-face.* Retrieved from https://campustechnology.com/articles/2018/06/18/most-students-say-online-learning-is-as-good-or-better-than-face-to-face.aspx

Schramm, W. (1962). What we know about learning from instructional television. In *Educational television: The next ten years.* Stanford, CA: The Institute for Communication Research, Stanford University.

Seaman, J. E., Allen, E., & Seaman, J. (2018). *Grade increase: Tracking distance education in the United States.* Retrieved from https://onlinelearningsurvey.com/reports/gradeincrease.pdf

Skiba, D. J. (2017, September/October). What has happened to massively open online courses? *Nursing Education Perspectives, 38*(5), 291–292. doi:10.1097/01.NEP.0000000000000222

Wetzel, D., Radtke, P., & Stern, H. (1994). *Instructional effectiveness of video media.* Hillsdale, NJ: Lawrence Erlbaum Associates.

Young, J. (2018, May). *Why the Lumina Foundation is betting big on new kinds of credentials.* Retrieved from https://www.edsurge.com/news/2018-05-15-why-the-lumina-foundation-is-betting-big-on-new-kinds-of-credentials

The Impact of New Directions on Teaching and Learning

Carol A. O'Neil and Cheryl A. Fisher

INTRODUCTION

A variety of factors are influencing the way we teach and the way we learn. Some include the changes in demographics and geographic characteristics of students enrolling in institutions of higher education, the financial considerations of traditional education, the advances in technology, and focus on career development. Delineating these factors and their impact on higher education is the focus of this chapter.

ENROLLMENT IN INSTITUTIONS OF HIGHER EDUCATION

Enrollment in institutions of higher education has been decreasing over the past several years. In 2016, 62% of students enrolled in institutions of higher education were in 4-year schools, 36% were in 2-year schools, and 2% enrolled in schools with less than 2-year programs (Ginder, Kelly-Reid, & Mann, 2017). Enrollment decreased nationally by 0.3% from spring 2017 to spring 2018 (National Student Clearinghouse Research Center, 2018), and specifically, enrollment in 4-year public institutions decreased by 0.9% during this past year, but enrollment in 2-year institutions is expected to stay the same (Hoover, 2017).

The decrease is most prevalent in 4-year institutions that are for profit (−6.8%), in 2-year public institutions (−2.4%), and in 4-year private (−0.3%) and nonprofit institutions (−0.4%). This is the pattern in 34 states and the Midwest and Northeast (National Student Clearinghouse Research Center,

2018). Elite institutions of higher education expect enrollment increases (Grawe, 2018).

The Council of Independent Colleges have held discussions about the status of enrollment in private liberal arts colleges. The identified issues included the potential burden of decreasing numbers of high-school graduates, the financial costs, and the competition among colleges for students. Possible solutions were changing the form of mergers and shifting of programs. The council decided that one change would not fit all schools and each school needs to make the changes that will best meet their individual needs (Seltzer, 2018).

First-time undergraduate student enrollment in fall 2016 increased in 37 states and the District of Columbia and decreased in the remaining states (Ginder et al., 2017). Students enrolling in online courses and programs are increasing. About 49% of students enrolled in online courses are at for-profit institutions; 18% of students enrolled in online courses are at nonprofit institutions; and 11% are in online courses at public institutions (Ginder et al., 2017). Almost 80% live locally and within 100 miles of their school (Magda & Aslanian, 2018). About 15% of students take an online course, and of these, 17% take both land-based and online courses (Seaman, Allen, & Seaman, 2018).

FINANCIAL IMPACT

College tuition is rising. Students and families rely on scholarship funds, loans, and savings to pay tuition. Approximately 47% of undergraduate and 64% of graduate students are employed and could be eligible for tuition reimbursement, yet at least 60% do not use employment reimbursement (Magda & Aslanian, 2018). Students tend to choose a school that awards scholarship funds over those that do not (Magda & Aslanian, 2018).

TECHNOLOGY

The Horizon Report is an annual analysis of the trends, challenges, and technologies that will drive education for the next 5 years (Becker et al., 2018). Measuring learning and redesigning learning space will be the focus in the next 1 to 2 years; open education resources and multidisciplinary learning will be the focus in 3 to 5 years; and the cultures of innovation and cross institution and cross sector collaboration will be the focus over the next 5 years and beyond (Becker et al., 2018). Solvable issues are providing authentic learning experiences and improving digital literacy. Issues that we understand, but do not know how to resolve, are adapting organizational designs to the future of work and advancing digital equity. Complex issues are economic and political pressures and rethinking the roles of educators (Becker et al., 2018).

Technology is a vehicle that teachers use to make decisions about technical and teaching strategies to effectively meet student-learning goals (Martin, 2018). One strategy is using mobile devices in teaching and learning. Over 80% of students use mobile devices for their online classes. They are accessing course material such as readings and course content, communicating with instructor and peers, and researching material for assignments (Magda & Aslanian, 2018). Gikas and Grant (2013) explored the use of mobile computing devices in higher education. They found that these devices allowed students to collaborate more effectively, which enhances engagement in communication and content creation. Educause Center for Analysis and Research (ECAR, 2017) surveyed tens of thousands of students across dozens of U.S. institutions to better understand student engagement with technology. Some of the key findings from this report noted that "laptops are king, smartphones are queen, and tablets are on the way out" (p. 5). The students identified their laptop as critical to their success, while three quarters identified their smartphone as moderately important, with the tablet functionality declining because it duplicates that of the laptop and smartphone. Another significant key finding noted that students would like instructors to use more technology in their classes, including lecture capture, early-alert systems, and search tools. These features were noted to be more desirable than features that require for the student to "give something" (p. 6) such as social media or polling tools.

Shadiev, Hwang, Huang, and Liu (2015) proposed integrating social media into conventional mobile learning to enhance collaboration through a system called m-learning. The aim of this system is to promote collaborative sharing of life experiences in nature and discussion of different perspectives. M-learning allows teaching and learning to expand beyond the traditional classroom with increased flexibility and opportunities for interaction. It is important to note that the successful integration of social media must come from a sound pedagogical approach attached to specific learning outcomes in order for this tool to be effective.

FOCUS ON CAREER DEVELOPMENT

Career development is the preparation of students for employment. We are currently in our third education revolution. The first was the expansion of high-school education. The second is the focus on associate degree programs, and this third revolution is lifelong learning.

The First Wave: The Expansion of High-School Education

The movement to enhance education through increased enrollment in high schools occurred from 1910 to 1940. The movement was strongest in the Midwest with the highest high-school enrollments in Iowa (Goldin & Katz, 1998), and by 1935, approximately 40% of youth earned a high-school diploma. The purpose of this high-school education was a response to economic changes through broadening education to enhance the preparation for employment (Selingo, 2018).

The Second Wave: The Growth of Associate Degree Programs

The Higher Education Act signed by Lyndon B. Johnson in 1965 paved the way for the expansion of post-high-school education. Enrollment in higher education increased and more than doubled between 1970 and 2016 (Selingo, 2018).

The Third Wave: Lifelong Learning

The first two waves focused on education at a young age and early in career development. This idea is changing to the view that education and training should be continuous through life owing to the impact of automation and the necessity for staying current and competent in evolving careers (Selingo, 2018). Staying competent in evolving careers means retraining in shorter periods rather than enrolling in degree programs. This retraining will come from two sources: employers supported and individual supported. Employers negotiate the retraining with their employees. There is an emerging group of freelance workers or contractors called the "gig economy." They are self-employed and must support their own training. This group will negotiate their own retraining (Selingo, 2018).

PREPARING STUDENTS FOR WORK

An ever-changing work environment results in graduates having outdated skills. Magda and Aslanian's (2018) survey of online students concluded that over three quarters of students registered for online courses that will enhance their careers and that they are seeking career services. Magda and Aslanian (2018) also found that 85% of students perceived education as a return on their investment. Employers tend to see the need for an innovation before educators are aware of them. When employers cannot initiate the needed innovation, friction results (Tishma, 2018). When educators focus on teaching the basic, most needed skills, the friction decreases, thereby resulting in employers and employees feeling more prepared for the work environment (Tishma, 2018). Employers report that maintaining the skills needed to perform a job is one of their top priorities.

Employers believe that the role of postsecondary education is to prepare students with the skills needed in their careers. In addition, a focus on "soft skills" should be provided. These are skills that will guide the student through the workplace after graduation and include critical thinking, resiliency, and communication (Arnett, 2018).

The literature supports a changing trend in the labor market due to technology. Trends in manufacturing are moving toward artificial intelligence and automation. In artificial intelligence and automation, machines complete tasks that have predictive patterns, such as driverless cars. Jobs lost to computerization can result in technological unemployment. Frey and Osborne (2013) studied the impact of these trends and found that 47% of the U.S. employment might be impacted by automation. A Gallup investigation at Northeastern University (Gallup Northeastern University, 2018) found that about 76% of those surveyed thought that artificial intelligence would impact their employment.

Jobs most likely influenced by artificial intelligence, called jobs with high automation risk, start at Point A and go to Point B. The functional tasks from point to point are predictable, thus allowing for the programming of machines to perform the tasks (Loeffler, 2018). Some of these jobs include telemarketing, retailing, administrative services, and transporting material (Frey & Osborne, 2013; Loeffler, 2018). Jobs at low risk for automation include organizational chief executives, recreational therapists, emergency management supervisors, creative and artistic workers, jobs requiring high levels of social intelligence, jobs requiring problem-solving and ingenuity, computer hardware engineers, mechanical engineers, and architects (Frey & Osborne, 2013; Loeffler, 2018). These jobs require social intelligence and problem-solving skills that are not yet amenable to programming a machine.

Most think that artificial intelligence and automation will make a positive difference but also think that jobs will be eliminated and retraining will be important. Most see this training as coming from their employer in the form of workshops and credentials (Gallup Northeastern University, 2018). However, this trend is creating a movement toward alternative learning environments that support creative and flexible ways to learn.

ALTERNATIVES TO VALIDATE LEARNING

One suggested flexible authentication of learning skills is competency-based education (CBE), which focuses on gaining competence rather than taking courses. Magda and Aslanian (2018) surveyed online students about CBE, and although students are more familiar with this approach, about 50% are interested and would like more information. Some institutions have combined the flexibility of an online CBE model with a project-based approach to real-world projects. One project-based CBE model was described by Ye, Van Os, Chapman, and Jacobson (2017) based on three value propositions: (a) identifying competencies that support program learning outcomes, (b) including project assignments that demonstrate mastery of competencies, and (c) coaching faculty to facilitate student performance in achieving mastery of competencies. With the growing demand for educators to prepare graduates for the work setting, work readiness has become a growing concern for employers. Once students have validated learning and demonstrated newly learned skills, they can earn certificates and combine them into stackable degrees. Magda and Aslanian (2018) surveyed online students and found that 95% were interested or very interested in the concept.

The stackable credential evolved over time from the part-time student taking one course at a time to eventually earning enough credits toward a degree. One of the problems with this approach is that taking courses for credit one at a time is inefficient; programs change in requirements over time, and they often do not map skills and competencies to a credential outcome (Jones-Schenk, 2018). Microcredentialing is a certification indicating a demonstrated competency in a specific skill. The new knowledge is not necessarily following a specific order or pathway but may generally fall into one of three models: vertical stacking, horizontal stacking, or value-added stacking (Hanover Research, 2017, p. 3). Vertical stacking refers to the more traditional method of stacking (or mapping) credentials into an academic credential or degree. Horizontal stacking is more about adding skills within a credential level. Value-added stacking focuses on adding skills or expertise for individuals who already hold an academic credential. These models have different applications for workforce development, both in developing new pipelines of workers and in developing expanded talent within incumbent workers. Today's stackable credential strategy attempts to combine the benefits of both the degree-related education and continuing education by mapping and stacking learning outcomes.

In the concept of textbook-free courses, textbooks are replaced with course material. Magda and Aslanian (2018) surveyed online students and found that about 50% of students are in favor of such an approach. As access to open resources continue to increase along with the cost of textbooks, textbook-free courses are becoming an attraction for many academic institutions. This approach allows for more opportunities for exploration and best practices and lessons learned from true experiences. Some of the reasons for movement in this direction include:

- The cost of textbooks for college students has increased 812% since 1978.
- The cost of course materials sometimes forces students to withdraw due to the additional financial burden.

Use of open educational resources (OER) allows faculty members to teach key concepts via lecture, ebook, and other means versus relying on reading concepts in a textbook. Some practical approaches can be used to design a course using video and other resources instead (Center for Teaching and Learning, 2016), for example, developing a set of learning resources, developing appropriate course assessments, fostering independent student exploration and research, and building on students' self-directed learning skills.

Although it may be difficult to think of a course without a textbook, new opportunities for exploration and application of content can now be considered.

THE IMPACT OF TECHNOLOGY

The impact of technology on education cannot be predicted, but educators cannot continue to exclusively teach using traditional methods. Educators must be agile, flexible, and responsive to the changing environment and needs of the learners (Hoover, 2017). Additionally, educators must be aware of the impact of technology on society and the changing needs of the learners. New opportunities continue to emerge for communication and collaboration in online classrooms, which has proven over time to be critical to learning. Technology is a powerful tool that can support and transform education in many ways, enabling new ways for people globally to work and learn together. Educators and instructional designers must work together to make the most of the opportunities provided by technology in order to continue making education efficient and available to everyone everywhere.

SUMMARY

With rapid change occurring in technical advancements from mobile devices to social media, educators have the opportunity and challenge to creatively design new educational environments that meet student needs. The rising cost of college degrees and textbooks have forced a shift in how future employees obtain education based on acquisition of skill. Employers themselves are looking for people ready to enter the workforce and participate in continued learning to maintain skill levels. All of these factors together have created a new way of looking at education which is taking on the shape of a traditional college education and continuing education.

REFERENCES

Arnett, A. (2018). *Preparing students for work required revised approach to education.* Retrieved from https://www.educationdive.com/news/preparing-students-for -work-requires-revised-approach-to-education/517738

Becker, S. A., Brown, M., Dahlstrom, E., Davis, A., DePaul, K., Diaz, V., & Pomerantz, J. (2018). *NMC horizon report: 2018 higher education edition.* Louisville, CO: EDU-CAUSE. Retrieved from https://library.educause.edu/~/media/files/library/ 2018/8/2018horizonreport.pdf

Center for Teaching and Learning. (2016). *Textbook-free courses.* Retrieved from https://ctl.learninghouse.com/textbook-free-courses

Educause Center for Analysis and Research. (2017). *ECAR study of undergraduate students and information technology, 2017.* Retrieved from https://library.educause. edu/~/media/files/library/2017/10/studentitstudy2017.pdf

Frey, C. B., & Osborne, M. A. (2013). *The future of employment: How susceptible are jobs to computerization.* Retrieved from https://www.oxfordmartin.ox.ac.uk/ publications/view/1314

Gallup Northeastern University. (2018). *Optimism and anxiety. Views on the impact of artificial intelligence on higher education's response*. Retrieved from https://www.northeastern.edu/gallup

Gikas, J., & Grant, M. M. (2013). Mobile computing devices in higher education. Student perspectives on learning with cellphones, smartphones and social medial. *The Internet and Higher Education, 19*, 18–26. doi:10.1016/j.iheduc.2013.06.002

Ginder, S. A., Kelly-Reid, J. E., & Mann, F. B. (2017). *Enrollment and employees in postsecondary institutions, fall 2016; and Financial statistics and academic libraries, fiscal year 2016: First look (provisional data) (NCES 2018-002)*. Washington, DC: National Center for Education Statistics, U.S. Department of Education. Retrieved from https://nces.ed.gov/pubs2018/2018002.pdf

Goldin, C., & Katz, L. (1998). *Human capital and social capital: The rise of secondary schooling in America, 1910 to 1940*. Cambridge, MA: The National Bureau of Economic Research. Retrieved from http://www.nber.org/papers/w6439

Grawe, N. D. (2018). *Demographic and demand for higher education*. Baltimore, MD: Johns Hopkins University Press.

Hanover Research. (2017). *Research brief: Stackable graduate credentials*. Arlington, VA: Author.

Hoover, E. (2017). Demographic changes as destiny in college admissions? It's complicated. *Chronicle of Higher Education*. Retrieved from https://www.chronicle.com/article/Demographic-Changes-as-Destiny/242062

Jones-Schenk, J. (2018). Alternative credentials for workforce development. Leadership and development. *Journal of Continuing Education in Nursing, 49*(10), 449–450. doi:10.3928/00220124-20180918-03

Loeffler, J. (2018). *The rise of AI and employment. How jobs will change to adapt*. Retrieved from https://interestingengineering.com/the-rise-of-ai-and-employment-how-jobs-will-change-to-adapt

Magda, A. J., & Aslanian, C. B. (2018). *Online college students. 2018. Comprehensive data on demands and preferences*. Louisville, KY: The Learning House. Retrieved from https://www.learninghouse.com/knowledge-center/research-reports/ocs2018/#cta-anchor

Martin, K. (2018). The key to 21st century classrooms isn't tech. It's evolved teaching. *EdSurge*. Retrieved from https://www.edsurge.com/news/2018-06-04-the-key-to-21st-century-classrooms-isn-t-tech-it-s-evolved-teaching

National Student Clearinghouse Research Center. (2018). *Current term enrollment estimates spring 2018*. Retrieved from https://nscresearchcenter.org/wp-content/uploads/CurrentTermEnrollment-Spring2018.pdf

Seaman, J. E., Allen, I. E., & Seaman, J. (2018). *Grade increase: Tracking distance education in the United States*. Retrieved from https://onlinelearningsurvey.com/reports/gradeincrease.pdf

Selingo, J. (2018). *The third education revolution*. Retrieved from https://www.theatlantic.com/education/archive/2018/03/the-third-education-revolution/556091

Seltzer, R. (2018). Small college struggles in the sights. *Inside Higher Ed*. Retrieved from https://www.insidehighered.com/news/2018/01/08/cic-presidents-institute-increases-focus-solutions-struggling-colleges

Shadiev, R., Hwang, W.-Y., Huang, Y.-M., & Liu, T.-Y. (2015). The impact of supported and annotated mobile learning on achievement and cognitive load. *Journal of*

Educational Technology & Society, 18(4), 53–69. Retrieved from https://www.jstor
.org/stable/jeductechsoci.18.4.53

Tishma, M. (2018). *On trend for 2018: Learning and flexibility.* Retrieved from http://
www.clomedia.com/2018/02/15/trend-2018-learning-flexibility

Ye, C., Van Os, J., Chapman, D., & Jacobson, D. (2017). An online project-based competency education approach to marketing education. *Journal of Marketing Education, 39*(3), 162–175. doi:10.1177/0273475317724843

3

Reflections on Pedagogy in Online Instruction

William A. Sadera and Kathleen A. Gould

INTRODUCTION

Pedagogy is the theory, methods, and activities for maximizing teaching and learning. Pedagogy of online learning includes employing active learning activities and interactivity that are essential for effective learning to take place. Pedagogy includes the consideration of the influence of learning theories upon which online learning environments are created. Without considering both current and historical pedagogical strategies, we risk losing opportunities to meet students' learning needs and the implementation of effective design. This chapter discusses research-based pedagogical approaches and their influence in online learning environments.

THE ADULT LEARNER

Online learners are often adults, and an effective instructor needs to understand how adults learn. Adults, compared to children and teens, have distinct needs and requirements as learners. Adult learning is not a unique and specific process. Instead, generalizations about "the adult learner" imply that people over a certain age form a homogeneous group. However, differences in culture, cognitive style, life experiences, and gender may be far more important to learning than age (Shannon, 2003).

Malcolm Knowles (1970) pioneered the field of adult learning and identified adult learning characteristics to include into the development of educational opportunities. Knowles found that adults are autonomous and self-directed. Teachers must actively involve adult participants in the learning process and serve as facilitators for them. Specifically, instructors must get the participants' perspectives about what topics to cover and let them work on projects that reflect their interests. Instructors should allow the participants to assume responsibility for presentations and group leadership. Instructors need to act as facilitators, guiding participants to their own knowledge rather than supplying them with facts. Finally, instructors must show participants how the class will help them reach their goals. Adults have accumulated a wealth of life experiences and knowledge that may include work-related activities, family responsibilities, and previous education. Adult learners need to connect learning to this knowledge and experience base. To help them do so, teachers should draw out the participants' experience and knowledge that is relevant to the topic. Effective educators relate theories and concepts to the participants and recognize the value of experience in learning.

Knowles also argued that adult learners are goal oriented. Upon enrolling in a course, adult learners usually know what goals they want to attain. These learners have an internally regulated desire to learn but also are concerned with ability comparisons, as are younger students (Remedios & Richardson, 2013). Therefore, they appreciate an educational program that is well organized and has clearly defined elements. Instructors must show participants how the class will help them attain their goals and must ensure that the course is relevant and practical. Learning should be applicable to their work or other responsibilities of value to them.

In adulthood, learning is optimized when the subject matter is presented in an authentic learning environment. Instructors must relate the relevance of the lesson to the learner's job or profession. Instructors must show adult learners respect and acknowledge the wealth of experiences these students bring to the classroom. Adult learners are equals in experience and knowledge and should be allowed to voice their opinions freely in class. Because of these characteristics, adult learning programs should capitalize on the experience of participants and should adapt to the age range of the participants. Additionally, the course offerings should consider advanced stages of participant development by offering as much choice as possible in the organization of the learning program.

CONSTRUCTIVISM

Constructivist learning is a pedagogical process oriented with an emphasis on collaboration and conversation among learners and teachers.

Often referred to as student centered, the constructivist approach to instruction is inductive progressing from the bottom up. Learning opportunities are diverse and increase in complexity. In this approach, the instructor is a model and a coach who encourages exploration of ideas, and learning is learner centered and learner generated. Constructivism is the process of bringing together new knowledge and experiences to construct a new reality and to make sense and meaning out of the world. Some teaching models include cognitive apprenticeship, minimalist training, intentional learning environments, and case- or problem-based instruction. These models lend themselves well to medical content and can be utilized to make learning meaningful. Other elements of this theory can be applied through design by:

- Allowing students to be responsible for their own learning
- Enabling students to manage their own learning activities
- Making maximum use of existing knowledge
- Anchoring instruction in realistic settings
- Providing multiple ways to learn content and express understanding
- Encouraging creative and flexible problem-solving

Constructivist educators believe that although the teacher imparts information, it does not necessarily mean that the student will learn. Constructivist educators believe that learning occurs when the learner synthesizes and makes sense of new information and connects the new information to existing understandings or schemas. Thinking inspires learning and is stimulated through activities. Active or experiential learning, according to Kolb (1984), involves the process of providing students with situations that require them to read, speak, listen, think, and create. Although lectures may be well written and well delivered, they often pass from the ear to the hand, leaving the mind untouched. The active learning process places responsibility on the learners themselves and lends itself to a wider range of learning styles.

Active learning online involves taking a critical look at the resources that already exist and incorporating them into the learning environment. Examples might include online discussion, vlogging, blogging, conferencing, or using wikis that would require learners to research information and then return to the online class environment to further collaborate and expand on their research findings. Technology can provide the richness that constructivist learning environments require to guide knowledge construction.

BEHAVIORAL THEORY

Behaviorism is based upon traditional beliefs about how we learn and is one of the most influential theories in the fields of education and psychology. Ivan Pavlov (1849–1936) conducted experiments in Russia with dogs. He rang a bell and then gave the dogs food. He repeated the ringing of the bell and the giving of food over and over until the dogs began to salivate in anticipation of food when the bell rang. This stimulus response behavior is called "classical conditioning." Edward Thorndike (1874–1949) applied behaviorism to education at Columbia University in New York. He postulated that learning was the resultant connection between a stimulus and a response. B. F. Skinner (1904–1990) continued to work with stimulus response but focused on studying voluntary responses. He rewarded responses that were desirable and punished or ignored undesirable responses. His work is called "operant conditioning." His theory, like those of Pavlov and Thorndike, was based on behavioral change, while mental processes were ignored. Behavioral change is what is observed—that is, what one says or does, or how one behaves. If a behavior is observed, it is the response to a stimulus. A stimulus is defined as an object in the environment that poses a physiologic threat. A response is anything that one does in response to a stimulus. It could be as simple as a turn of the head, a twitch, or saying "I am sorry" or as complex as designing a building or writing a book. Behaviorism was popular until the 1950s, but it began to lose supporters because the theory explained learning from only a behavioral perspective and is therefore limited in scope. The psychological theory of behaviorism is used as an educational theory when the learning experience is based on a stimulus and a response, and by rewarding behavior that will meet the educational goal and ignoring (or correcting) behavior that is not goal directed. In behavioral theory, large tasks are broken down into smaller tasks, and each task is learned in successive order. The process is called "successive approximations." Behaviorist-based instructional practice is usually teacher centered and designed around the instructor presenting information and the students passively receiving that information and presenting the knowledge they acquired back to the instructor for assessment. Traditional learning labs are an example of behaviorist theory. In this environment, a student may be learning the correct procedure for a dry, sterile dressing. Using behavioral practices, the instruction is focused on taking the entire procedure and breaking it down into steps: Learners master the first step and then move to successive steps until they master every step to complete the procedure. In the preceding example, the first steps would be to verify the order, then gather equipment, and then prepare the client, set up the area for a sterile field, and so forth. By learning a segment at a time and doing each segment correctly, the student will be able to successfully complete the dry, sterile dressing procedure by putting the learned steps together.

SOCIAL INTERACTION

Social interaction has long been thought to increase collaboration and, therefore, result in increased learning. Jung, Choi, Lim, and Leem (2002) studied interactions in groups and learning outcomes and concluded that adult learners who engaged in social interaction with their instructors and collaborative interaction with peers scored higher on outcome measures of learning than adult learners who did not engage in social and collaborative interaction. Diep, Cocquyt, Zhu, and Vanwing (2016) studied factors that influenced online participation and found that educational levels predicted discussion contribution with those who had achieved a higher level of education being less likely to contribute. Employment status predicted collaborative facilitation with those having full-time or part-time employment being more likely to collaborate than full-time students. Finally, female gender and higher educational status were associated with greater social interaction in online discussions (Diep et al., 2016). This interaction continues to be recognized as one of the most important components of learning experiences in both conventional education and distance education (Bacalarski, n.d.). In fact, Jonassen (2013) argued that technology should be utilized to "support social negotiation and construction of knowledge" (p. 108).

Interaction has less to do with personal interaction (e.g., building a community of learners) and more to do with providing a means of reinforcing various elements from the content of the training (Cahill, 2014). Research has shown that learning in groups improves students' achievement of learning objectives. Vygotsky (1978) argued that cognitive development and learning are dependent on social interaction. The major theme of his theoretical framework is that social interaction plays a fundamental role in the process of learning. A second aspect of Vygotsky's theory is the idea that the potential for cognitive development is limited to a certain "time span," which he refers to as the zone of proximal development (ZPD). It is during this time that consciousness is raised, and a range of skills can be developed with adult guidance or peer collaboration. Vygotsky's methods of analysis and conclusions about the development of human thought and language are still well regarded today and can be applied to the study of computer-mediated communication (Bacalarski, n.d.). Online learning allows for the use of various tools that encourage communication, collaboration, and the exchange of ideas between learners. This interaction allows the learner to consider additional perspectives and critically evaluate their assumptions as they construct knowledge (Cahill, 2014). Given the potential interactive nature of online learning environments and the needs of adult learners, the connections between these theories and this population are self-evident.

PROBLEM-BASED LEARNING

Problem-based learning (PBL) is an instructional method that involves the presentation of a clinical problem as a teaching strategy (Ridley, 2007). Donner and Bickley (1993) described PBL as a form of education that allows for information to be mastered in the same context in which it is used. PBL, because of its ability to provide an authentic problem as the stimulus for learning, fulfills the requirements of a cognitive apprenticeship as described by Brown, Collins, and Duguid (1989).

PBL has the characteristics of a constructivist, student-centered learning environment as advocated by Jonassen (2000). In this environment, learners are provided with a question, issue, case, project, or problem that they attempt to solve. The PBL process is structured in four specific phases. Phase one involves students reasoning through the problem and identifying their learning needs in groups. The next phase consists of learners engaging in self-directed learning as they explore the topic. In phase three, the group process takes over with each learner applying the results of individual research to the problem. Finally, the fourth phase involves the summary of the information gathered and utilization of this information in problem-solving (Neville, 2009). PBL, because of its ability to elicit problem-solving and critical analysis, endeavors to bridge the gap between theoretical knowledge and practical application. Medical schools in the United States began utilizing PBL in the 1970s, and since then it has become commonplace. More recently, PBL has been incorporated as a teaching method in the education of other health professionals, including nurses, physical therapists, and public health professionals.

Learners are assisted in their pursuit of knowledge by an instructor who has more expertise in the area than the learners themselves. In line with constructivist approaches to learning, the instructor facilitates, but does not direct or dictate, learning. Learning is accomplished independently but is greatly supported by the participation of the instructor who provides guidance in the discovery process. The learners also benefit from the preexisting knowledge and research shared by other group members in pursuit of problem resolution. Woltering, Herrler, Spitzer, and Spreckelsen (2009) found that medical students using online PBL had an increased motivation for learning and higher satisfaction with their learning gains over students in the traditional PBL environment. The online support of the PBL process had benefits for the students and resulted in improved cooperation. King et al. (2010) studied online PBL in an interprofessional health sciences course and found that the online learning environment facilitated small group collaborative interactions. Conducting PBL online could be advantageous to increasing discipline-specific skills, team skills, and fluency with information technology.

The online environment allows students to utilize a variety of resources beyond traditional textbooks to pursue self-directed learning, an essential feature of PBL. Hill, Wiley, Nelson, and Han (2004) argued that "learning with" Internet resources allowed students to actively construct something unique as they used the Internet for information gathering. Internet resources utilized in this manner become "cognitive tools" that enhanced human thinking, problem-solving, and learning. Bozic and Williams (2011) found that students enjoyed the flexibility of PBL and the opportunity to promote reflection. Specifically, students preferred the ability to gather information at their own pace to reflect on and construct solutions to problems. The variety of online resources available also helped support individual learning styles.

PBL can improve students' critical-thinking skills and motivation for learning and enhance student autonomy and self-direction. Furthermore, PBL increases students' ability to apply their learning to practice and enables them to use a variety of resources to pursue learning. These features of PBL can enable students to become more effective practitioners and lifelong learners.

SUMMARY

Pedagogy is the practice of teaching and provides frameworks and theories for effective teaching and learning. A theory comprises constructs and concepts that are put into action, thus operationalizing the theory into practice. The theories in this chapter were adult learning theory, constructivism, behaviorism, social interaction, and PBL. Adult learning theory characterizes the adult learner as knowledgeable and experienced, preferring to work on topics that interest them. They are goal oriented and responsible for their learning. This type of learning differs from constructivist theory, which is process oriented and student centered. Knowledge is reinforced through active learning. Behaviorism focuses on stimulus and response in which action that meets the objective is reinforced. Social interaction learning is based on participation and discussion. PBL is based on authentic learning that is the outcome of engaging in problem-solving activities. Applying the concepts of one of these theories in planning learning allows for predictability of the learning process that contributes to learning.

REFERENCES

Bacalarski, M. C. (n.d.). *Vygotsky's developmental theories and the adulthood of computer mediated communication: A comparison and an illumination.* Retrieved from http://psych.hanover.edu/vygotsky/bacalar.html

Bozic, N., & Williams, H. (2011). Online problem-based and enquiry-based learning in the training of educational psychologists. *Educational Psychology in Practice, 27*(4), 353–364. doi:10.1080/02667363.2011.590466

Brown, J., Collins, A., & Duguid, P. (1989). Situated cognition and the culture of learning. *Educational Researcher, 18*(1), 32–42. Retrieved from http://www.aera.net/publications/?id=317

Cahill, J. (2014). How distance education has improved adult education. *The Educational Forum, 78*(3), 316–322. doi:10.1080/00131725.2014.912366

Diep, N., Cocquyt, C., Zhu, C., & Vanwing, T. (2016). Predicting adult learners' online participation: Effects of altruism, performance expectancy, and social capital. *Computers & Education, 101*(1), 84–101. doi:10.1016/j.compedu.2016.06.002

Donner, R., & Bickley, H. (1993). Problem-based learning in American medical education: An overview. *Bulletin of the Medical Library Association, 81*(3), 294–298. Retrieved from http://www.ncbi.nlm.nih.gov/pmc/articles/PMC225793

Hill, J. R., Wiley, D., Nelson, L. M., & Han, S. (2004). Exploring research on Internet-based learning: From infrastructure to interactions. In D. H. Jonassen (Ed.), *Handbook of research for educational communications and technology* (2nd ed., pp. 433–460). Mahwah, NJ: Lawrence Erlbaum Associates.

Jonassen, D. H. (2000). Revisiting activity theory as a framework for designing student-centered learning environments. In D. H. Jonassen & S. M. Land (Eds.), *Theoretical foundations of learning environments* (pp. 89–122). Mahwah, NJ: Lawrence Erlbaum Associates.

Jonassen, D. H. (2013). Transforming learning with technology. In M. P. Clough, J. K. Olson, & D. S. Niederhauser (Eds.), *The nature of technology* (pp. 101–112). Rotterdam, Netherlands: Sense Publishers.

Jung, I., Choi, C., Lim, C., & Leem, J. (2002). Effects of different types of interaction on learning achievement, satisfaction, and participation in web-based instruction. *Innovations in Education and Teaching International, 39*(2), 153–162. doi:10.1080/14703290252934603

King, S., Greidanus, E., Carbonaro, M., Drummond, J., Boechler, P., & Kahlke, R. (2010). Synchronous problem based e-learning (e-PBL) in interprofessional health science education. *Journal of Interactive Online Learning, 9*(2), 133–150. Retrieved from http://www.ncolr.org/jiol/issues/pdf/9.2.3.pdf

Knowles, M. (1970). *The modern practice of adult education: Andragogy versus pedagogy.* New York, NY: The Association Press.

Kolb, D. A. (1984). *Experiential learning: Experience as the source of learning and development* (Vol. 1). Englewood Cliffs, NJ: Prentice-Hall.

Neville, A. J. (2009). Problem-based learning and medical education forty years on: A review of its effects on knowledge and clinical performance. *Medical Principles and Practice, 18*(1), 1–9. doi:10.1159/000163038

Remedios, R., & Richardson, J. (2013). Achievement goals and approaches to studying: Evidence from adult learners in distance education. *Distance Education, 34*(3), 271–289. doi:10.1080/01587919.2013.835776

Ridley, R. (2007). Interactive teaching: A concept analysis. *Journal of Nursing Education, 46*(5), 203–209. Retrieved from https://www.healio.com/journals/jne/2007-5-46-5/%7B216fcec7-1fb1-484a-85e9-575dc4502248%7D/interactive-teaching-a-concept-analysis

Shannon, S. (2003). Adult learning and CME. *The Lancet, 361*(9353), 266. doi:10.1016/S0140-6736(03)12262-3

Vygotsky, L. (1978). *Mind in society: The development of higher psychological processes.* Cambridge, MA: Harvard University Press.

Woltering, V., Herrler, A., Spitzer, K., & Spreckelsen, C. (2009). Blended learning positively affects students' satisfaction and the role of the tutor in the problem-based learning process: Results of a mixed-method evaluation. *Advances in Health Science Education, 14*, 725–738. doi:10.1007/s10459-009-9154-6

4

Flexible Learning Environments

Shannon Tucker and Matthew J. Rietschel

INTRODUCTION

The concept of flexible learning environments in traditional classrooms has been applied to learning since the inception of movable furniture in a classroom. At its core, flexible learning environments are intended to change the focus of the learning from teacher led to a facilitator-guided, student-centered one. The most fundamental structures in an educational setting are often the barriers to progress: mandatory schedules, physical spaces, grouping of learners, and use of human capital (Jacobs & Alcock, 2017).

The three main principles of flexible learning environments include those of environment, learner grouping, and how the instructional time is programmed. The first began with the ability to augment the physical space, floor plans, and furniture choices. The idea grew into the environment to the use of flexible grouping for students (i.e., reading and math levels) to how time is used in flexible methods throughout the educational time. These three main principles are now being applied to the online learning environment. Technology plays a central role in the development of flexible online learning environments by providing tools that enable instructors to bridge distance, time, and other physical barriers that persist in traditional educational environments. Examples of the specific technologies are presented in Chapter 10, Technical Considerations to Support Learning Environments.

Although the discussions of learning theories in Chapter 3, Reflections on Pedagogy in Online Instruction, are pragmatic, the exploration of the learning theories and frameworks in this chapter is presented in a conceptual manner. The content is presented in this fashion to highlight the key constructs that influence flexible learning environments. This chapter is not intended to be inclusive of all frameworks and learning theories but rather highlights three concepts that fundamentally support the need and foundational underpinnings for flexible learning environments. Technological pedagogical content knowledge (TPACK) framework is included to highlight the intersection of the concepts, and each profoundly augments the other and is not simply an add-on to an existing concept. The framework provides a clear groundwork to build a flexible learning environment, as it addresses the environment, technology, content, and learners. Cognitive theory of multimedia learning (CTML) is incorporated to understand the impact and effective use of multimedia learning. The use of multimedia is a logical choice, as it quickly and efficiently reaches many different types of learners and areas of content. Finally, the chapter explores the universal design for learning (UDL), which must be part of the conversation when discussing flexible learning environments.

TPACK FRAMEWORK

Viewed through the TPACK framework (Figure 4.1), effective teaching with technology thoughtfully integrates subject-matter expertise and content-appropriate pedagogical practice with technology in a given educational context (Koehler & Mishra, 2009). TPACK builds on Shulman's (1986) concept of pedagogical content knowledge (PCK), recognizing the reciprocal influence technology, content, and pedagogy have on teaching practice (Koehler & Mishra, 2009; Mishra & Koehler, 2006). In this context, technology integration is not simply layering technology on top of existing teaching practice; its weight is equal to content and pedagogy. As seen in the intersection of content knowledge (CK), pedagogical knowledge (PK), and technological knowledge (TK), the TPACK construct provides a way to think about the construction of learning environments that considers the context and conditions that surround online learning.

Description of Intersections

CK represents the subject-matter knowledge of an instructor (Mishra & Koehler, 2006). Unique between disciplines, instructor expertise in the conceptual knowledge, related theories, and content-appropriate

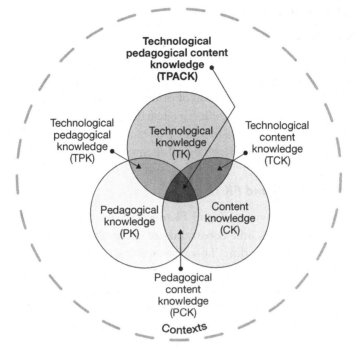

FIGURE 4.1 The components of TPACK.

practices for learning knowledge development is critical (Mishra & Koehler, 2006; Shulman, 1986).

PK represents the knowledge of effective teaching practice (Koehler & Mishra, 2009; Mishra & Koehler, 2006). This includes theoretical and practical knowledge related to learner development of knowledge and expertise, educational theory and practice, course planning and management, and learner assessment (Koehler & Mishra, 2009). Expertise in this area contributes to the use of practices that result in both effective learning and positive learner experiences (Koehler & Mishra, 2009).

TK represents fluency in technology use and the appropriate application of technology to solve problems or achieve goals (Koehler & Mishra, 2009). Although CK and PK development may lead to an "end state" where critical knowledge development is achieved, no such state is achieved with TK, as technology is in a continuous state of development requiring continuous development as changes impact daily life and practice (Koehler & Mishra, 2009).

TPACK Constructs

Intersection of CK and PK

The relationship between CK and PK draws from Shulman's (1986) ideas about the pedagogical adaptation of subject matter as they interpret content for instruction. Consideration of prior knowledge, content-area misconceptions and application, effective teaching practice, and assessment are factors that must be considered by instructors when creating a flexible learning environment (Koehler & Mishra, 2009).

Intersection of TK and PK

The relationship between TK and PK necessitates instructors to understand the affordances and constraints of technology as they relate to teaching practice, including how the application of technology may support or limit teaching practice (Koehler & Mishra, 2009). In online teaching environments, this is a critical consideration given that technology tool selection in online environments is not always the domain of an instructor. Although school or campus adoption of learning management systems (LMSs), web conferencing, and other collaboration tools provides ubiquitous access to technology tools, eliminating licensing and access constraints for instructors, it also standardizes the technology-based constraints that must be considered when adopting pedagogical practices in online environments.

Intersection of TK and CK

The relationship between TK and disciplinary CK is seen in our understanding of the world around us. Advances in technology have fundamentally changed the practice of astronomy, medicine, neuroscience, and physics, where the use of technology has changed our understanding of the discipline and disciplinary knowledge has shaped our use of technology (Koehler & Mishra, 2009). This extends to our use of technology in education to teach subject-matter content in online environments where discipline-specific CK influences the selection and use of technology and technology affordances influence the practices of CK development. As a result, instructors must balance content importance and technology affordances toward content-related learning goals with an aim to enhance the learner development of CK by maximizing the affordances technology offers (Koehler & Mishra, 2009).

Intersection of TK, PK, and CK

Koehler and Mishra (2009) situate TPACK as a professional knowledge construct that necessitates fluency in technology, pedagogy, and content and their interrelationships. This provides a foundation for effective teaching with technology, allowing instructors to evaluate how to best represent concepts with technology, how technology and pedagogies can work together for a meaningful learning experience, and how technology can help support student success in learning difficult content (Koehler & Mishra, 2009; Mishra & Koehler, 2006). Although TPACK has faced criticism for oversimplifying the nuances of each key domain, the model's simplicity allows instructors to focus on their own teaching context, allowing the development of solutions that are context appropriate (Graham, 2011; Koehler & Mishra, 2009; Mishra & Koehler, 2006). This assumes that instructors are well versed and comfortable in their knowledge of key domains and constructs to design effective, pragmatic solutions (Koehler & Mishra, 2009).

TPACK Example

When TPACK is used effectively, it is a meaningful interlacing of the three types of knowledge and the instructor's purposeful use of a specific technology (TK) to improve student learning (PK) in a specific learning context (CK). An example in present-day nursing programs is the use of the electronic health record (EHR) in practice. The instructor designs a learning activity that accounts for the student's knowledge of the EHR technology (how to functionally use it and why to do so) and their nursing CK, and then the instructor chooses a pedagogical approach that supports this content and the objective of the activity.

COGNITIVE THEORY OF MULTIMEDIA LEARNING

In online learning environments, multimedia instruction may take the form of online lectures or videos, simulations, demonstrations, web conferences, or LMS-embedded learning modules. Broadly defined as a presentation with words and pictures (Mayer, 2009), multimedia is used as an umbrella term to classify a variety of presentation forms. Although CTML does not recognize individual differences in capacity between the auditory and visual channels or neuroplasticity in learners (Rose &

Meyer, 2006), it does provide a framework to consider the relationship between multimedia design principles and learner cognitive processing (Mayer, 2005, 2009).

Cognitive Processes Associated With Multimedia Learning

By depicting the processing of words (visual and auditory) and pictures in two channels through the memory system, CTML synthesizes prior research in cognitive function, providing a shorthand to discuss learning with multimedia (Mayer, 2009). CTML's three assumptions—dual channel assumption, limited capacity assumption, and active processing assumption—provide a foundation to understand the impact multimedia design has on learner cognitive processing (Mayer, 2003). This then supports the use of multimedia design principles to manage the cognitive load of learners.

Assumptions Associated With CTML

1. Dual Channel Assumption

    Learner information processing is conducted in two independent channels: an auditory (or verbal) channel and a visual (or pictorial channel; Mayer, 2005, 2009). As learners view a multimedia presentation, word (written or verbal) and pictures (images/video) are processed into the auditory (ears) and visual (eyes) channels within sensory memory (Figure 4.2; Mayer, 2005, 2009).
2. Limited Capacity Assumption

    The limited capacity assumption states that learner auditory and visual channels have a limited capacity for sensory input (Mayer, 2005, 2009). The limited cognitive capacity of visual and auditory information learners can hold and reference in working memory results in selective attention and the application of compensatory metacognitive strategies (Mayer, 2009).
3. Active Processing Assumption

    Learners undergo an active learning process to integrate existing knowledge in long-term memory with new knowledge in working memory (see Figure 4.2; Mayer, 2005). Learners actively adopt mental models to assimilate and accommodate new information, creating a new coherent model (Mayer, 2009). Information from working memory and long-term memory intersect as learners'

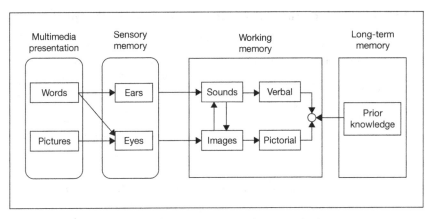

FIGURE 4.2 Cognitive theory of multimedia learning.

Source: Reproduced with permission from Mayer, R. E. (2005). Cognitive theory of multimedia learning. In R. E. Mayer (Ed.), *The Cambridge handbook of multimedia learning* (pp. 31–48). Cambridge, UK: Cambridge University Press.

active cognitive processes select relevant information, organize information coherently, and integrate connections with prior knowledge (Mayer, 2009).

MULTIMEDIA DESIGN IN PRACTICE

The assumptions associated with CTML provide a basis for the development of practical design principles aimed at improving learning with multimedia. The design principles for effective multimedia design, given in Table 4.1, provide specific guidance to reduce extraneous processing associated with poor instructional design, manage essential processing by helping learners process complex information more effectively, and foster generative processing by helping motivate student engagement (Mayer, 2009, 2011; Mayer & Fiorella, 2014).

However, it is important to note the limitations of CTML. Although CTML provides a simplified structure for dual channel processing of auditory and visual elements (Baddeley, 1986; Paivio, 2007) and cognitive load theory (Baddeley, 1986; Sweller & Chandler, 1991), CTML does not directly recognize the differences in cognitive capacity or neuroplasticity (Rose & Meyer, 2006), raising questions regarding the boundary conditions that limit the effectiveness of these multimedia design principles.

TABLE 4.1   Design Principles for Effective Multimedia Design

	Design Principle	Approach
Principles to Reduce Extraneous Processing	Coherence	Eliminate irrelevant and unnecessary text or graphics to focus attention
	Signaling	Provide cues, arrows, or highlights to emphasize essential information
	Redundancy	Limit use of verbatim text in default onscreen presentation*
	Spatial Contiguity	Place corresponding words/graphics in close proximity
	Temporal Contiguity	Show corresponding words/graphics simultaneously
Principles to Manage Essential Processing	Segmenting	Segment presentations to allow learner control over the pace of the unit
	Pretraining	Present key concepts and vocabulary before or at the beginning of a presentation
	Modality	Use narration in presentations with printed text and graphics
Principles to Foster Generative Processing	Multimedia	Use relevant text and explanatory graphics rather than text alone
	Personalization	Where appropriate, use a conversational language to make the presentation more relatable
	Generation Principle	Ask or encourage students to self-test, diagram/draw concepts, or write key information to engage with content
	Voice	Do not use computer-generated narration/voices

*This does not apply to closed captioning.

UNIVERSAL DESIGN FOR LEARNING

By combining cognitive neuroscience and the architectural design concept, universal design (UD), UDL guides the design of inclusive and flexible learning environments that create meaningful learning experiences for all learners (Rose & Meyer, 2006). UDL promotes the development of outcomes, instructional methods, adoption of materials, resources, and student assessments to create flexible environments aimed at reducing barriers to learning (Center for Applied Special Technology [CAST], 2011; Meyer, Rose, & Gordon, 2014). Based on the concept of neurovariability and neuroplasticity, UDL's guidelines align instructional design with evidence-based practices for inclusive learning.

THE VARIABLE LEARNER

Neuroplasticity is a concept where by the neural networks form and change synaptic connections in the brain in response to the environment (Kaas, 2001). Seen in normal brain development and repair following brain injury, neuroplasticity is an essential component in learning (CAST, 2018a; Kaas, 2001; Meyer et al., 2014). This plasticity can be seen in thousands of neural pathways, resulting in infinite variations of brain pathways between learners (CAST, 2018a; Meyer et al., 2014). However, the complexity of brain anatomy makes it difficult to digest all the brain systems associated with learning. Focusing on broad networks associated with memory, language, problem-solving, and thinking provides a broad perspective on learning (Rose & Strangman, 2007). Addressing the role of the recognition, affective, and strategic network classes of the brain, UDL helps simplify cognitive neuroscience into a spatially distinguishable system to think about learning holistically (Meyer et al., 2014; Rose & Strangman, 2007). This provides a scientifically based mechanism to support the predictable needs of learners (Meyer et al., 2014).

Affective networks are central to learner engagement and moderate learner motivation, interest, effort, persistence, and ability to self-regulate in learning activities (CAST, 2018a; Meyer et al., 2014; Rose & Strangman, 2007). Located in the center of the brain, affective networks are the "why" of learning (Meyer et al., 2014). Ultimately, affective networks shape how learners engage in learning environments (CAST, 2018a). This is seen in learners' response to difficult tasks and their persistence in the face of adversity or disengagement when the task seems like an insurmountable obstacle (Rose & Strangman, 2007).

Recognition networks are key to processing what we see, hear, taste, touch, and smell into recognizable patterns (Meyer et al., 2014; Rose & Strangman, 2007). Located in the back of the brain, the recognition networks are the "what" of learning (Meyer et al., 2014). Essential to higher level cognitive function, recognition networks are central to perception, pattern recognition, language, symbol decoding, and overall comprehension (CAST, 2018a; Rose & Strangman, 2007). In learning, recognition networks effect what learners perceive, remember, and comprehend when faced with problems (Rose & Strangman, 2007).

Strategic networks moderate our actions and expressions in learning environments (Meyer et al., 2014). Located in the frontal lobe area of the cortex, strategic networks help learners perform tasks by planning, organizing, self-monitoring, and executing both physical and cognitive actions (Meyer et al., 2014; Rose & Strangman, 2007). Closely associated with executive function, strategic networks are the "how" of learning, moderating all of our actions (CAST, 2018a; Meyer et al., 2014).

UDL PRINCIPLES

Using neuroscience as a basis to predict the needs of learners, UDL provides a mechanism to support learner variability without individualizing instruction (CAST, 2018b; Meyer et al., 2014). The foundational principles of UDL provides a way for educators to scaffold effective practices systematically.

Principle: Provide Multiple Means of Engagement

Shaped by the affective network, the ways learners are motivated and engaged in learning are unique based on their experience (CAST, 2018b). At its core, this principle aims to provide multiple means for learners to engage based on their interest, ability to sustain effort, and self-regulate learning (CAST, 2018b; Meyer et al., 2014). Checkpoints provide a guide for instructors to ensure that their environment supports student engagement (Table 4.2; CAST, 2018b).

Principle: Provide Multiple Means of Representation

Although sensory, cognitive, and learning disabilities are commonly understood as affecting learner perception, learner comprehension varies systematically based on past experiences, knowledge, culture, and their understanding of language being used (Meyer et al., 2014). UDL checkpoints for representation (Table 4.3) help instructors

TABLE 4.2   Guidelines for Engagement

Guideline	Checkpoint
Recruiting Interest	Optimize choice and autonomy Optimize relevance, value, and authenticity Minimize threats and distractions
Sustaining Effort and Persistence	Heighten salience of goals and objectives Vary demands and resources to optimize challenge Foster collaboration and community Increase mastery-oriented feedback
Self-Regulation	Promote expectations that optimize motivation

TABLE 4.3   Guidelines for Representation

Guideline	Checkpoint
Perception	Offer ways of customizing the display Offer alternatives for auditory information Offer alternatives for visual information
Language and Symbols	Clarify vocabulary and symbols Clarify syntax and structure Support decoding of text, mathematics, and symbols Promote understanding across languages Illustrate through multiple media
Comprehension	Activate or supply background knowledge Highlight patterns, critical features, big ideas, and relationships Guide information processing and visualization Maximize transfer and generalization

ensure sensory, language, and comprehension is supported in a way that allows learners to customize their learning experience without necessitating individual accommodation (CAST, 2018b).

Principle: Provide Multiple Means of Action and Expression

Learners approach tasks differently depending on their physical and strategic/organizational abilities (CAST, 2018b; Meyer et al., 2014; Table 4.4). UDL guidelines for physical action, expression and communication, and executive function support learner participation to ensure that they can appropriately access material and participate equally (CAST, 2018b).

TABLE 4.4   Guidelines for Action and Expression

Guideline	Checkpoint
Physical Action	Vary methods for response and navigation Optimize access to tools/assistive technologies
Expression and Communication	Use multiple forms of media for communication Use tools that support construction and composition Build fluency with graduated levels of support for practice
Executive Function	Guide goal setting Support planning and strategy development Facilitate managing information and resources Enhance capacity for monitoring progress

UDL IN PRACTICE

In health science disciplines in which learners are required to possess specific physical and sensory abilities and language requirements for the successful completion of professional tasks and procedures to complete a program, the application of UDL may seem contradictory. Yet, grounded in evidence-based practice, the UDL framework provides a structure that supports the infinite variation of learners who participate in online learning environments by both maximizing cognitive capacity and providing a framework that can be flexibly adapted to the learner's experiences and environment.

Keeping learners engaged is a serious concern in online learning (Bawa, 2016). It is unclear how motivation and other social factors contribute systematically to retention rates (Bawa, 2016; Chen & Jang, 2010). However, ensuring learning environments are able to capitalize on student interest, support persistence, and maximize self-regulation, keeping students motivated and engaged with learning is key. Although additional research is needed to assess the effect of UDL's engagement principle on learner retention in online environments, early research shows a positive influence on students' intention to participate and usefulness of learning (Al-Azawei, Parslow, & Lundqvist, 2017). By intentionally focusing on engagement principles, instructors can avoid design decisions that may inadvertently discourage students and contribute to attrition.

Considering the construction of learning objects, UDL's perception guideline is compatible with the principles of CTML when CTML is used to inform the creation of content for use in visual and auditory learning objects. However, in ensuring learners with sensory disabilities have equal access to content, UDL helps ensure learners have flexible access to content that meets their environmental or technology limitations. Instead of having one way to access content, learners with technical issues still have an opportunity to access material without instructor intervention. Similarly, learners are free to select content formats that work within environmental constraints, where one format of content may be impractical or impossible to see or hear despite a learner's sensory abilities (e.g., listening to audio while commuting/driving, reading while in a waiting room, etc.), creating an environment that responds to the emergent needs of learners seamlessly.

In practice, UDL's reach extends from the design and construction of learning environments to the instructional design of activities within them. Although instructors may not need to be concerned that a campus LMS is accessible and provides the necessary functions to support sensory and physical disabilities, attention is needed to leverage these functions to provide a flexible experience for learners that benefits the spectrum of learner variability both seen and unseen.

SUMMARY

This chapter described how the learning theories and frameworks can be applied to create a flexible learning environment. The chapter began with a description of TPACK to underscore how the intersection of the different paradigms combine to form something that is more than the sum of its parts. The remainder of the chapter discusses the concept of designs that ensure that learning is consumable by the surfeit of learners, content, and technology. Although the chapter intends to provide a foundation to the frameworks/theories that should be considered when designing a flexible learning environment, it does not provide practical application of them. The following chapters expand upon the process of reconceptualizing, practical application, management, and technical considerations.

REFERENCES

Al-Azawei, A., Parslow, P., & Lundqvist, K. (2017). The effect of universal design for learning (UDL) application on e-learning acceptance: A structural equation model. *The International Review of Research in Open and Distributed Learning, 18*(6). doi:10.19173/irrodl.v18i6.2880

Baddeley, A. D. (1986). *Working memory*. Oxford, England: Oxford University Press.

Bawa, P. (2016). Retention in online courses: Exploring issues and solutions—A literature review. *Sage Open, 6*(1). doi:10.1177/2158244015621777

Center for Applied Special Technology. (2011). *Universal design for learning guidelines version 2.0*. Retrieved from http://udlguidelines.cast.org

Center for Applied Special Technology. (2018a). *UDL and the learning brain*. Retrieved from http://www.cast.org/our-work/publications/2018/udl-learning-brain-neuroscience.html

Center for Applied Special Technology. (2018b). *The UDL guidelines*. Retrieved from http://udlguidelines.cast.org

Chen, K. C., & Jang, S. J. (2010). Motivation in online learning: Testing a model of self-determination theory. *Computers in Human Behavior, 26*(4), 741–752. doi:10.1016/j.chb.2010.01.011

Jacobs, H. H., & Alcock, M. (2017). *Bold moves for schools: How we create remarkable learning environments*. Alexandria, VA: ASCD.

Kaas, J. H. (2001). Neural plasticity. In N. J. Smelser & P. B. Baltes (Eds.), *International encyclopedia of the social & behavioral sciences* (pp. 10542–10546). Amsterdam, The Netherlands: Elsevier. doi:10.1016/B0-08-043076-7/03619-6

Mayer, R. E. (2003). The promise of multimedia learning: Using the same instructional design methods across different media. *Learning and Instruction, 13*(2), 125–139. doi:10.1016/S0959-4752(02)00016-6

Mayer, R. E. (2005). Cognitive theory of multimedia learning. In R. E. Mayer (Ed.), *The Cambridge handbook of multimedia learning* (pp. 31–48). Cambridge, England: Cambridge University Press.

Mayer, R. E. (2009). *Multimedia learning* (2nd ed.). Cambridge, UK: Cambridge University Press.

Mayer, R. E. (2011). Applying the science of learning to multimedia instruction. In J. P. Mestre & B. H. Ross (Eds.), *Psychology of learning and motivation* (Vol. 55, pp. 77–108). San Diego, CA: Elsevier Academic Press.

Mayer, R. E., & Fiorella, L. (2014). Principles for reducing extraneous processing in multimedia learning: Coherence, signaling, redundancy, spatial contiguity, and temporal contiguity principles. In R. E. Mayer (Ed.), *The Cambridge handbook of multimedia learning* (2nd ed., pp. 279–315). New York, NY: Cambridge University Press. doi:10.1017/CBO9781139547369.015

Meyer, A., Rose, D. H., & Gordon, D. (2014). *Universal design for learning: Theory and practice*. Wakefield, MA: Center for Applied Special Technology.

Paivio, A. (2007). *Mind and its evolution: A dual coding theoretical approach*. Mahwah, NJ: Lawrence Erlbaum Associates.

Rose, D. H., & Meyer, A. (Eds.). (2006). *A practical reader in universal design for learning*. Cambridge, MA: Harvard Education Press.

Rose, D. H., & Strangman, N. (2007). Universal design for learning: Meeting the challenge of individual learning differences through a neurocognitive perspective. *Universal Access in the Information Society, 5*(4), 381–391. doi:10.1007/s10209-006-0062-8

Sweller, J., & Chandler, P. (1991). Evidence for cognitive load theory. *Cognition and Instruction, 8*(4), 351–362. doi:10.1207/s1532690xci0804_5

TPACK REFERENCES

Graham, C. R. (2011). Theoretical considerations for understanding technological pedagogical content knowledge (TPACK). *Computers & Education, 57*(3), 1953–1960. doi:10.1016/j.compedu.2011.04.010

Koehler, M. J., & Mishra, P. (2009). What is technological pedagogical content knowledge (TPACK)? *Contemporary Issues in Technology and Teacher Education, 9*(1), 60–70. Retrieved from https://www.citejournal.org/volume-9/issue-1-09/general/what-is-technological-pedagogicalcontent-knowledge/

Mishra, P., & Koehler, M. J. (2006). Technological pedagogical content knowledge: A new framework for teacher knowledge. *Teachers College Record, 108*(6), 1017–1054. doi:10.1111/j.1467-9620.2006.00684.x

Shulman, L. S. (1986). Those who understand: Knowledge growth in teaching. *Educational Researcher, 15*, 4–14. doi:10.3102/0013189X015002004

5

Guiding Structures for New Learning Environments

Cheryl A. Fisher and Carol A. O'Neil

INTRODUCTION

Guiding structures are entities that exist in the environment and serve as guideposts to creating, configuring, implementing, and evaluating online learning environments. Guiding structures are modalities of online teaching and learning arranged or rearranged into new systems or structures. One guiding structure for online teaching and learning is interaction and communication that connects the learners with each other, the learners with the content, and the learner with the faculty facilitator. Other guiding structures related to the learners are learning style and learning generations. Learning style impacts how a student best learns, such as some learners like listening to lectures, others like reading, and some learn by doing. The generation of the learner influences the way he or she best learns. An example is that Baby Boomers are computer learned and not computer natives because they did not have computers in home or school during their formative years. Generation Z remembers always having computers at home and in school and a phone in their pockets. Technology guides some of the guiding structures such as adaptive learning in which student responses in learning environment guides the next step in the learning process or mobile learning in which learners download apps to their phone to enhance or guide the learning process. Learning modalities, such as massive open online courses (MOOCs), certificates, microcredentials, and stackable certificates/degrees, allow for flexible lifelong learning environments. Information and impact of these

47

guiding structures follow. This chapter provides an overview of pertinent considerations when designing and teaching online courses.

GUIDING PRINCIPLES FOR COMMUNICATING ONLINE

Instructional interactivity and communication take place among the instructor, the learner, and the content (Figure 5.1), and they are included in the instructional design plan. In a traditional classroom, communication between the teacher and the student and among students is generally synchronous (occurring at the same time and place). In distance learning, communication can be either synchronous or asynchronous (not occurring at the same time). When faculty and students interact and engage in the face-to-face classroom, they develop intellectual and personal relationships. Interaction between learners and online content is the strongest predictor of student satisfaction, and learning and online courses include activities that strengthen the interactions (Lin, Zheng, & Zhang, 2017).

IMPORTANCE OF INTERACTION

A successful online course is easy to access and easy to navigate. Interactivity means more than just clicking a mouse button to advance to the next page. Interactivity requires meaningful feedback (i.e., leading toward an established goal) for each learner. Purposes for providing online discussion include providing an open question-and-answer forum, encouraging critical thinking, achieving social interaction and community building, validating experiences, and supporting student reflections and inquiries (Pendry & Salvatore, 2015). Often, this involves written response, called a dialogue with the instructor or other learners. In the online environment, interaction can take place in the form of a question-and-answer session or a discussion and may be asynchronous or synchronous. Moore (1993) described three types of interaction that are critical to student learning in the online environment: (1) learner to content, (2) learner to instructor, and (3) learner to learner. Learner-to-learner interaction is important as it can take place in the form of group activities or group discussion forums (Figure 5.1). Since Moore's (1993) seminal work, an additional type of interaction has been identified between the learner and the interface, which is providing an essential

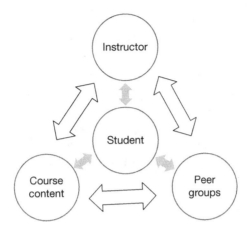

FIGURE 5.1 Elements of interaction in online learning environments.

means of interaction with the content, instructor, and other learners. The student's experience with the interface can lead to student dissatisfaction if the technology is not user friendly (Cho, 2011).

The characteristics of a "good" online conversation includes evidence of problem-solving, informed decision-making, and depth of both student and teacher in facilitated discussions. The conversation should extend beyond a simple question-and-answer interaction to the examination of complex problems from multiple perspectives. The environment design should facilitate and promote critical thinking, knowledge expansion, and opportunities for students to draw from their experiences. Questions that encourage exploration and research might include Socratic-type probing, such as the following:

- What leads you to think that?
- What is your reasoning?
- What are the alternative strategies?
- From your experiences, did you find this to be the case?
- Expand on what you mentioned in your post.

Effective social constructivist learning uses interactive online discussion and Socratic questioning. These models of collaborative learning are essential in course design and delivery as online learning strategies in a quality online course.

Students describe feelings of isolation in online courses. Interaction allows students the opportunity to meet their peers and share ideas and experiences, thus reducing isolation. Dziuban et al. (2015) studied interaction and found that quality learning is largely the result of ample interaction with the faculty, other students, and content. Lieberman (2018) views group work on a continuum of disequilibrium of effort between higher achieving students and those who do not put in as much effort to influencing productive collaboration and idea sharing. A characteristic of a "good" teacher is one who is knowledgeable and proficient about the content. Learner–instructor interaction provides students with access to expert faculty and thus enhances satisfaction of the learning experience.

INSTRUCTOR-TO-STUDENT INTERACTIONS

Instructor and student interaction is an important aspect for student learning in an online course (Pendry & Salvatore, 2015). The tasks of the course facilitator are to ensure that what the student shares is correct. The facilitator contributes information, experiences, references, and stories that validate student learning and enhance discussions.

STUDENT-TO-CONTENT INTERACTIONS

In traditional environments, textbooks, PowerPoint slideshows, and video clips make up the instructional content for a class. In distance courses, instructors decide how to deliver course content along with the guidance of an instructional designer. More sophisticated delivery modes are becoming popular as increased bandwidth and fiber optics allow for the downloading of multimedia files, such as PowerPoint, Flash, or YouTube presentations (with or without associated audio), and streaming video. However, the instructor should not convert materials used in traditional courses without considering how distance technologies allow for the efficient and effective use of the course materials. Additionally, the instructor needs to consider whether the students are able to access multimedia requiring plug-ins for viewing and to access large data files. Reducing files into smaller sizes (i.e., a text version of an audio file) allows the students to have options for accessing course information based on preference. Depending on how the technology is used, students may find it easier to use or interact with distance learning content than with traditional classroom content. Instructor notes or slides available for print from the course site allow students to take notes more thoroughly while listening to online lectures. The material is accessible to students at their convenience. This material includes animated graphics that create simulations to demonstrate blood flow or actions of the cranial nerves and help students visualize body processes better than a one-dimensional textbook is capable of showing.

STUDENT-TO-STUDENT INTERACTIONS

Student-to-student interaction using asynchronous communication (not simultaneous or concurrent in time) can take place in the main discussion area of an online course or in collaborative groups. One of the main challenges of online education is providing methods and tools for interaction that takes advantage of technology's unique features such as the use of discussion boards. Discussion boards can offer benefits including reflection, analysis, and higher-order thinking (AlJeraisy, Mohammad, Fayyoumi, & Alrashideh, 2015). The main discussion area of an online course should be analogous to the main classroom in a face-to-face course. This discussion area is where the students and the instructor meet to participate in active dialogue and discuss course material and where students have the opportunity to learn from each other and ask questions for further understanding of course content. Interaction is an important component of the online learning dynamic, and technology is responsible for bringing students together. For more information and examples of student activities, see the Illinois Online Network website: www.ion.uillinois.edu/resources/otai/index.asp.

GROUP COLLABORATION

Groups or learning teams are another means by which the instructor can promote collaboration and interaction in the online classroom. Instructional activities and assignments that provide students with a variety of ways to engage each other have a direct and immediate effect on student performance (Stephens & Roberts, 2017). When the instructor builds in a variety of activities and experiences, online course work is more engaging and effective. This allows students to work through concepts, brainstorm, and work together. Building in options and opportunities for students to work together or individually is highly recommended. Groups or teams can be especially effective when working on case scenarios or problem-based learning (PBL) activities. Students can self-select group membership, or the instructor can assign students to groups. Sometimes students like to work together based on experience. Post guidelines and expectations of team performance. For example:

- Each team will designate, elect, or appoint a team coordinator or leader.
- The leader will remain the same throughout the course unless replaced by a majority vote of the team or by the instructor.
- The team leader may make a decision unless overruled by a majority.
- Any project assigned to the group will receive a grade that applies to every member of that group.
- The team leader will have the opportunity for input regarding any team member's grade.
- The instructor will have the final say in all cases in which the team cannot reach a decision.

Team members will evaluate each other's work, participate, and contribute to the team assignment. Team self-evaluation is an option to offer teams to help promote a productive work environment. For example, the instructor might ask:

1. What worked?
2. What needed improvement?
3. How would you make these improvements?

SYNCHRONOUS COMMUNICATION

Synchronous communication can take place in the form of Skype or other interactive videoconferencing. The greatest challenge of synchronous communication or meetings is to coordinate a time when all participants are available. Considerations are differences in time zones, students working different shifts, and the hardware requirements (i.e., webcam and microphone).

The logistics of timing live meetings can truly be reason enough not to use them. If students are working shifts in different time zones, it may be impossible to find a time that is convenient for all. Nurses working the night shift may have to get up in the middle of the day to participate. This will lead to reduced quality in their contributions and disruption in sleep prior to going back to work. When students are international, the window for meeting times is further reduced.

In the online environment, Internet meeting using web cameras is an option, but this technology works best for a small number of individuals. Synchronous videoconferencing or webinars require students to be at a certain place at a certain time. Possibilities for actual participation in lectures offered in remote places exist, but they may require that the student visit a campus or other location that has the videoconferencing technology in place. This technology allows students in several locations to share the same learning experience simultaneously through two-way video and audio.

BUILDING COMMUNITY

Regardless of the type of communication, students should feel as if they are a part of the learning community. Distance students often feel isolated and alone in their early experiences online, but with proper guidance and personalized attention, they quickly bond and come to depend on each other for learning and moral support. One strategy for instructors to use to begin building community is an initial request for posting of a biography. The instructor can model how to post a "bio" by posting one first and asking for (1) professional experiences, (2) educational background, and (3) personal information within the student's comfort level. The bios will allow students to find commonalities and provide the opportunity to get to know each other. Another technique may be to use icebreakers. Online or virtual icebreakers can include games or strategies to get students to know each other and to get the conversations flowing. These icebreakers allow students to seek others in the class with similar interests or experiences that may facilitate positive working relationships and problem-solving. Another strategy for facilitating community is to set up a chat or a student lounge area where students can meet and greet without loading up the main classroom with personal chatter.

Social software can show a human face online and help students and faculty communicate, educate, and interact with their communities. These software tools include blogs, wikis, social networking software, photo sharing, podcasting, and more. They are easy to use and popular and thus have potential for tremendous impact on learning. It is important to require alignment of the task and the technology to obtain the most benefit and a seamless integration of the tool into learning.

ACTIVE LEARNING

Engaging in active learning activities facilitates the meaning-making process that is a part of the constructivist approach. Learners relate their life experience and knowledge to the context of the online classroom. In nursing, for example, students use case-based scenarios or problems to analyze nursing issues. The online instructor promotes active learning through the creative use of instructional design strategies. For example, the incorporation of web quests or PBL scenarios will facilitate meaningful active learning and help students search for real-life answers. A web quest is an inquiry-oriented activity in which some or all of the information that learners interact with comes from resources on the Internet (Dodge, 1997). Web quests can be of either short or long duration, and they are intentionally designed to make the best use of a learner's time. Web quests should contain at least the following components:

- The introduction orients students and captures their interest.
- The task describes the activity's end product.
- The process explains strategies students should use to complete the task.
- The resources are the websites students will use to complete the task.
- The evaluation measures the results of the activity.
- The conclusion sums up the activity and encourages students to reflect on its process and results.

Information sources might include web documents, experts who are available via email or web conferencing, searchable online databases, books, and other documents physically available to the learner. Several examples of nursing web quests are available on the web. One example is a web quest that provides nursing students with an activity related to exploring the concepts of chronic illness and the impact on patients and families (see questgarden.com/137/38/1/111222124351/index.htm).

PBL using case-based scenarios is another example of active learning strategies that promote collaboration among teams of students. PBL is an instructional method that challenges students to "learn to learn," working cooperatively in groups to seek solutions to real-world problems. These problems engage students' curiosity and initiate learning the subject matter. PBL prepares students to think critically and analytically and to find and use appropriate learning resources. With its roots in the medical profession, PBL was originally developed to assist interns to determine a diagnosis based on the given symptoms of a patient. PBL promotes student initiative as a driving force and supports a system of student–faculty interaction in which the student assumes primary responsibility for the process (Neville, 2009).

Cognitive apprenticeship is a strategy that involves close communication between experts and novices in an authentic context. Nurses taking clinical courses in community health, adult health, or other practical areas will need to be involved in this type of learning experience. In this environment, novices progress along a path to expertise by refining authentic products and processes under the mentorship of experts. Cognitive apprenticeships are within the social constructivist paradigm and suggest that students work in teams on projects or problems. They are representative of Vygotski's "zones of proximal development" in which student tasks are slightly more difficult than students can manage independently, requiring the aid of their peers and instructor to succeed (Brown, Collins, & Duguid, 1989).

As with any apprenticeship, this involves observation of experts in action, coaching of novices by experts, and successive approximation to expert work as novices gain expertise. The students may be physically present in a hospital or community to develop skills while participating in the didactic part of the course online. Ongoing dialogue and conversations between and among students and instructors will help students to identify problems that they may encounter or skills that they need to develop.

Interaction and communication has been identified as the core of the course where learning takes place in an online environment. The interaction among instructors, students, and the course content is necessary to apply content and develop knowledge.

GENERATIONS AND LEARNING STYLES

Principles of adult learning, learning styles, and generational differences influence learning. In planning education and training, educators can affect learning through an analysis of this information. The recognition of learning styles and teaching based on that recognition will help faculty and instructional designers to create more efficient and effective methods of teaching.

According to Knowles, Holton, and Swanson (2015), andragogy characterizes the principles of adult learning based on six assumptions:

1. Need to know: Adults must understand why they need to learn new information.
2. Self-concept: Adults are responsible for their own lives and are self-directed.
3. Role of the learners' experiences: Adults draw upon learners' experience as it relates to new education.
4. Readiness to learn: Adults learn concepts they need to use.
5. Orientation to learning: Adults are life centered or problem centered.
6. Motivation: Internal pressures (self-esteem, quality of life) are higher motivators to learning than external motivators (job and salary) are.

With learning, adults need more focus on the entire process rather than teaching on specific content. A variety of teaching strategies capture participants' learning styles. Visual, auditory, and kinesthetic learning styles are the most prevalent. In addition to learning styles, generational differences among learners play a role in how adults learn.

Baby Boomers were born between 1946 and 1964. Their characteristics are that they tend to be dependent on education to obtain information. They learn best in a caring environment with positive feedback. They want to know the "what" and "how" and then the "why" prior to learning, and they are process oriented. Baby Boomers learn best by lectures and talk time and prefer individual to group work. Generation X was born between 1965 and 1980. This generation comprises independent problem solvers who multitask. They are concrete thinkers and technology literate. They find that technology is a necessity, and they learn through trial and error. They enjoy fun, interactive simulations, and mentoring by the older generations.

The generation of students referred to as the Generation Y or millennials has grown up using technology including smartphones, messaging, social networks, email, and blogs and regards technology as essential in all parts of their lives including learning. This millennial generation includes those typically born between 1981 and 1999. Millennials grew up in an era when technology, instant communication, and social networking are second nature. Texting, cell phones, MP3 players, CDs, and DVDs are at their fingertips, and text messaging is their primary method of communication (Phillips, 2016). This engagement in technology has created some distinct characteristics in the way in which these generations communicate and learn. Millennials have had technology embedded in their lives from an early age and exhibit distinct learning preferences such as teamwork, experiential activities, structure, instant feedback, and seamless technology integration. Many exhibit a short attention span demanding quick and easy access to relevant, bite-sized information in real time through online search engines, social networks, and online company repositories. Millennials prefer less structured forms of learning and more collaboration with peers. Group-based projects that emulate the work environment (authentic assessments) are ideal for these learners, including "googling" and discovery of information. Laskaris (2015) described the five Rs of millennial learning preferences that influence learning, and they are research based, relevance, rationale, relaxed, and rapport. The millennials are more likely to engage with learning content that is audio, video, and kinesthetic and prefer less lecture and more collaboration. They are expert at finding web-based information and respond positively when given the rationale behind policy and procedure-based information. Millennials thrive in learning environments that allow time for learning, are more relaxed, and respond well when given positive and personal acknowledgment from the instructor. Mentors and mentorship are also features that millennials are looking for in current educational and work settings.

Generation Z follows the Gen Xers and has similar learning characteristics and preferences for learning based on their upbringing in a technical world. Generation Z includes those born from 1995 to around 2012 (Turner, 2015); however, authors disagree on exact Generation Z cutoff dates. Similar to Generation X, Generation Z grew up completely immersed in technology from iPads to smartphones. They are referred to as the iGeneration, Gen Tech, Net Gen, or digital natives with their primary means of communication being text messaging. To date, the research continues as to their learning needs and differences from the millennials.

ADAPTIVE LEARNING

"Adaptive learning," in the most general terms, can be defined as a way of delivering learning materials online, in which the learner's interaction with previous content determines the nature of materials delivered subsequently. The process is automated, dynamic, and interactive. Its purpose is to generate a personalized learning experience. Adaptive learning can help students take ownership in their learning. For example, an adaptive quizzing system was implemented as a strategy to support student persistence and performance measured by use, grades, and graduation rates. Results indicated that use of the system increased course content mastery and predicted final course grades. Adaptive quizzing is efficient and helps focus on how each student's learning of content was tailored to his or her estimated ability level (Newman, Stokes, & Bryant, 2013). Within the adaptive quiz system, a student's ability level is determined and continuously updated based on responses to calibrated questions. As students answer more difficult questions correctly, they are given increasingly more challenging questions on subsequent quizzes. As they answer the more challenging questions correctly, students move up in their ability to master the content.

MOBILE LEARNING TECHNOLOGY

As mobile devices continue to connect us across the globe, it seems evident and unavoidable that universities and learning environments integrate them into wireless networks for mobile learning. University campuses and higher education continue to focus on learner centered mobile learning offering students increased opportunities for access to learning content. The term mobile learning (m-learning) refers to the use of mobile and handheld IT (information technology) devices, such as personal digital assistants (PDAs), mobile telephones, laptops, and tablet PC (personal computer) technologies (Alsaadat, 2017) for the purpose of accessing and studying learning materials and communicating with fellow students and instructors. The advantage of mobile learning is the convenience offered to the learner. There is a significant absence of attention, however, to pedagogical details in conceptualizing m-learning. Although m-learning is attractive to learners, the use of mobile technology does not guarantee that effective learning will occur. Without reference to theoretical and pedagogical issues, studies of m-learning will not necessarily further our understanding of how m-learning can contribute to successful learning outcomes globally (Al-Zahrani & Laxman, 2016).

MASSIVE OPEN ONLINE COURSES

First introduced in 2006, MOOCs are free online courses available for anyone to enroll. MOOCs provide an affordable and flexible way to learn new skills, advance careers, and obtain quality educational experiences. Originally, the purpose of MOOCs was to increase enrollment in participating universities. However, that has not been the case. The format of the MOOCs consisted of large discussion groups with peers, streaming video lectures, and multiple choice questions and quizzes. This format was nothing new from a pedagogical viewpoint. This is what is known about MOOCs:

- The number of MOOCs increased by 2,000 in the last year.
- The average number of MOOCs offered by the top U.S. News & World Report universities increased from 12 to 17.
- The top 50 U.S. News universities offer 26 more MOOCs than the bottom 50.
- The growth in the number of MOOCs results from an increased number of international universities now offering these courses.
- The rate of MOOC completion is low at 7% to 12%.
- MOOCs have been successful in providing students all over the world access to a wide range of subjects from world-renowned universities.

MOOCs allow learners to create their own learning pathway, thereby building upon their own prior learning and experiences. The typical student enrolled in a MOOC, according to Schaffhauser (2017), is a male in his 20s from outside the United States seeking a certificate. MOOC students are heterogeneous in their backgrounds with computer science and other science, technology, engineering, and math (STEM) courses demonstrating the largest enrollment. Schaffhauser (2017) also found that there has been steady enrollment in MOOCs. There is a slight decrease in combining the MOOCs into certificates because of current charges for this service.

MICROCREDENTIALING AND CERTIFICATES

Microcredentialing (digital badging) is the process of earning a microcredential, a minidegree or certification, in a specific topic area. They can be broad in topic such as nursing management or may be more specific. To earn a microcredential, you would need to complete a certain number of activities, assessments, or projects related to the topic. Once the requirements are completed, the credential is awarded. Although still largely undefined, microcredentials are competency based and provide evidence of mastery of a skill learned. Digital badges—awarded by institutions, organizations, groups, or individuals—recognize a particular experience or signify accomplishments, such as completion of a project or mastery of a skill. Badging documents skills gained through various learning and engagement opportunities via professional organizations and communities. These digital credentials are recognizing ongoing learning that can include service, leadership, and subject-matter expertise.

As badging lacks standards and varies widely in requirements, the concern is how to determine the value of a badge. The value in each badge is dependent on the credibility of the issuer and the badge requirements. Other concerns include the risk to an issuer's brand if a badge earner does not perform as expected. Senior campus administrators may be hesitant to endorse a badging program if it resides outside the academic program or lacks appropriate oversight for the assessment of learning outcomes. As an emergent and rapidly evolving field, criteria for credible badges must align with competency frameworks or educational standards within specified professions. Badging has the potential to change the way we think about professional development and lifelong learning as learning does not stop when we achieve a degree or a new position. Badges signify a professional achievement and ongoing professional development to colleagues and to a current or prospective employer. As the field of badging evolves, badges will align with competencies and skills directly applicable in the workplace, and training programs will use badges in ways that can support advancement along a career pathway.

SUMMARY

This chapter described the well-documented importance and the types of interaction for learning that occur in online environments. The guiding principles for communicating online described the differences and advantages in using synchronous and asynchronous communication and the importance of developing communities of learning. As online courses continue to increase and learners evolve from Baby Boomers to Generation Z, the impact of technology on the learner continues to be a factor needing consideration in course design. And finally, the traditional

2- or 4-year college degree is now challenged by new systems involving badges and microcertificates providing participants with education and skills as opposed to just knowledge.

REFERENCES

AlJeraisy, M., Mohammad, H., Fayyoumi, A., & Alrashideh, W. (2015). Web 2.0 in education: The impact of discussion board on student performance and satisfaction. *The Turkish Online Journal of Educational Technology, 14*(2), 247–258. Retrieved from http://www.tojet.net/articles/v14i2/14227.pdf

Alsaadat, K. (2017). Mobile learning technologies. *International Journal of Electrical and Computer Engineering, 7*, 2833–2837. doi:10.11591/ijece.v7i5.pp2833-2837

Al-Zahrani, H., & Laxman, K. (2016, Spring). A critical meta-analysis of mobile learning research in higher education. *Journal of Technology Studies*. Retrieved from https://scholar.lib.vt.edu/ejournals/JOTS/v42/v42n1/al-zahrani.html

Brown, J. S., Collins, A., & Duguid, P. (1989). Situated cognition and the culture of learning. *Educational Researcher, 18*, 32–42. doi:10.3102/0013189X018001032

Cho, T. (2011). The impact of types of interaction on student satisfaction in online courses. *International Journal on E-Learning, 10*(2), 109–125. Retrieved from https://www.learntechlib.org/p/32381

Dodge, B. (1997). *Some thoughts about webquests.* Retrieved from http://webquest.org/sdsu/about_webquests.html

Dziuban, C., Moskal, P., Thompson, J., Kramer, L., DeCantis, G., & Hermsdorfer, A. (2015). Student satisfaction with online learning: Is it a psychological contract? *Online Learning, 19*(2), 10–13. doi:10.24059/olj.v19i2.496

Knowles, M. S., Holton, E. F., & Swanson, R. A. (2015). *The adult learner. The definitive classic in adult education and human resource development* (8th ed.). Oxon, England: Routledge.

Laskaris, J. (2015). How to engage millennials: 5 important moves. *eLearning*. Retrieved from https://www.efrontlearning.com/2016/03/5-strategies-to-engage-the-mil lennials.html

Lieberman, M. (2018). *Online students do not have to work solo.* Retrieved from https://www.insidehighered.com/digital-learning/article/2018/04/25/group-projects -online-classes-create-connections-and-challenge

Lin, C. H., Zhang, Y., & Zheng, B. (2017). The role of learning strategies in online language learning: A structural equation modeling analysis. *Computers & Education, 113*, 75–85. doi:10.1016/j.compedu.2017.05.014

Moore, M. (1993). Theory of transactional distance. In D. Keegan (Ed.), *Theoretical principles of distance education* (pp. 22–38). New York, NY: Routledge.

Neville, A. J. (2009). Problem-based learning and medical education forty years on. A review of its effects on knowledge and clinical performance. *Medical Principles and Practice, 18*(1), 1–9. doi:10.1159/000163038

Newman, A., Stokes, P., & Bryant, G. (2013). *Learning to adapt: A case for accelerating adaptive learning in higher education.* Boston, MA: Education Growth Advisors.

Pendry, L., & Salvatore, J. (2015). Individual and social benefits of online discussion forums. *Computers in Human Behavior, 50*, 211–220. doi:10.1016/j.chb.2015.03.067

Phillips, M. (2016). Embracing the multigenerational nursing team. *Medsurg Nursing*, 25(3), 197–200.

Schaffhauser, D. (2017, January 12). Harvard/MIT report analyzes 4 years of MOOC data. *Campus Technology*. Retrieved from https://campustechnology.com/articles/2017/01/12/harvard-mit-report-analyzes-4-years-of-mooc-data.aspx

Stephens, G., & Roberts, K. (2017). Facilitating collaboration in online groups. *Journal of Educators Online, 14*(1). Retrieved from https://www.thejeo.com/archive/2017_14_1/stephens_roberts

Turner, A. (2015). Generation Z: Technology and social interest. *The Journal of Individual Psychology, 71*(2), 103–113. doi:10.1353/jip.2015.0021

6

Reconceptualizing the Online Learning Environment

Carol A. O'Neil

INTRODUCTION

Reconceptualizing is the process of making decisions about learning content that will be organized for an online learning environment. A program can be reconceptualized into courses, courses can be reconceptualized into modules, and modules can be reconceptualized into headings (topics).

RECONCEPTUALIZING A PROGRAM

Pedagogy, infrastructure, and technology form the foundation for the decision tree found in Figure 6.1. Reconceptualizing a program is answering questions in the decision tree and using the answers to guide the development of online learning environments. The decision tree is a series of "if–then" statements that comprise questions, possible answers, and possible actions. Questions relate to the characteristics of the institution, technology, faculty, and students. Possible answers to the questions are given, and actions based on each of the possible responses are proposed.

The following is an example of using a decision tree to guide decision-making. A school of nursing is considering moving their RN to BSN program online. The school has a strategic plan, developed with input from faculty that includes online learning. This information about institutional factors leads to the conclusion that support for online programs

Institutional Issues

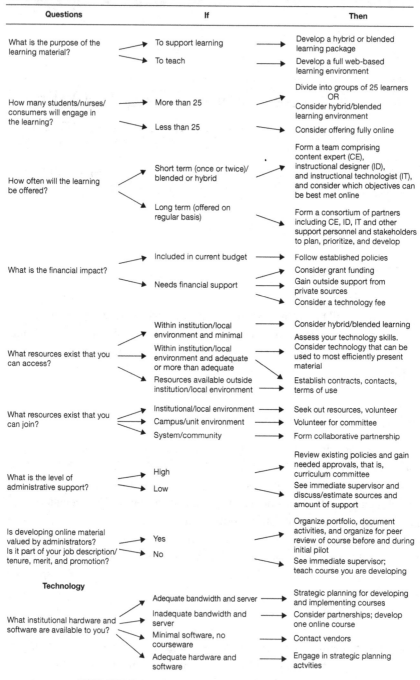

Questions	If	Then
What is the purpose of the learning material?	To support learning	Develop a hybrid or blended learning package
	To teach	Develop a full web-based learning environment
How many students/nurses/consumers will engage in the learning?	More than 25	Divide into groups of 25 learners OR Consider hybrid/blended learning environment
	Less than 25	Consider offering fully online
How often will the learning be offered?	Short term (once or twice)/blended or hybrid	Form a team comprising content expert (CE), instructional designer (ID), and instructional technologist (IT), and consider which objectives can be best met online
	Long term (offered on regular basis)	Form a consortium of partners including CE, ID, IT and other support personnel and stakeholders to plan, prioritize, and develop
What is the financial impact?	Included in current budget	Follow established policies
	Needs financial support	Consider grant funding
		Gain outside support from private sources
		Consider a technology fee
What resources exist that you can access?	Within institution/local environment and minimal	Consider hybrid/blended learning
	Within institution/local environment and adequate or more than adequate	Assess your technology skills. Consider technology that can be used to most efficiently present material
	Resources available outside institution/local environment	Establish contracts, contacts, terms of use
What resources exist that you can join?	Institutional/local environment	Seek out resources, volunteer
	Campus/unit environment	Volunteer for committee
	System/community	Form collaborative partnership
What is the level of administrative support?	High	Review existing policies and gain needed approvals, that is, curriculum committee
	Low	See immediate supervisor and discuss/estimate sources and amount of support
Is developing online material valued by administrators? Is it part of your job description/tenure, merit, and promotion?	Yes	Organize portfolio, document activities, and organize for peer review of course before and during initial pilot
	No	See immediate supervisor; teach course you are developing
Technology		
What institutional hardware and software are available to you?	Adequate bandwidth and server	Strategic planning for developing and implementing courses
	Inadequate bandwidth and server	Consider partnerships; develop one online course
	Minimal software, no courseware	Contact vendors
	Adequate hardware and software	Engage in strategic planning actvities

FIGURE 6.1 Reconceptualizing the online course.

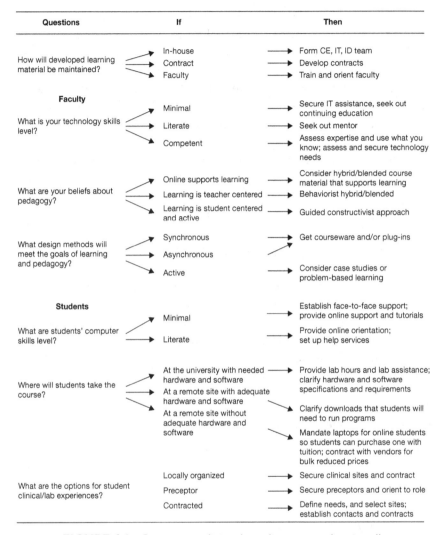

Questions	If	Then
How will developed learning material be maintained?	In-house	Form CE, IT, ID team
	Contract	Develop contracts
	Faculty	Train and orient faculty
Faculty		
What is your technology skills level?	Minimal	Secure IT assistance, seek out continuing education
	Literate	Seek out mentor
	Competent	Assess expertise and use what you know; assess and secure technology needs
What are your beliefs about pedagogy?	Online supports learning	Consider hybrid/blended course material that supports learning
	Learning is teacher centered	Behaviorist hybrid/blended
	Learning is student centered and active	Guided constructivist approach
What design methods will meet the goals of learning and pedagogy?	Synchronous	Get courseware and/or plug-ins
	Asynchronous	
	Active	Consider case studies or problem-based learning
Students		
What are students' computer skills level?	Minimal	Establish face-to-face support; provide online support and tutorials
	Literate	Provide online orientation; set up help services
Where will students take the course?	At the university with needed hardware and software	Provide lab hours and lab assistance; clarify hardware and software specifications and requirements
	At a remote site with adequate hardware and software	Clarify downloads that students will need to run programs
	At a remote site without adequate hardware and software	Mandate laptops for online students so students can purchase one with tuition; contract with vendors for bulk reduced prices
What are the options for student clinical/lab experiences?	Locally organized	Secure clinical sites and contract
	Preceptor	Secure preceptors and orient to role
	Contracted	Define needs, and select sites; establish contacts and contracts

FIGURE 6.1   Reconceptualizing the online course. (*continued*)

is strong. The dean is willing to provide information technology (IT) and instructional design (ID) support. The program will enroll more than 25 students and will be long term. The current budget will support development and maintenance activities for faculty and learning.

The school has 3-year-old desktop computers for faculty members. Several laptops are available to faculty and all computers have Internet access. Computer laboratories are available for students, with over 50 terminals in the school of nursing with Blackboard access available.

Faculty members who are computer literate and have experience teaching online are available and willing to teach the courses. There are faculty orientation and development programs for online teaching available to faculty. Expertise of students is varied and there is learning material for online students to orient them to online learning. The decision made based on the characteristics of the answers to the "if–then" statements was to move the program online. The RN to BSN program would be developed starting with two courses a semester.

Another possible scenario that might exist is high technical support and minimal faculty skill. If the faculty is motivated and willing to learn to develop online courses, develop the course online. If there is moderate support and high resources, develop the course online. If there is minimal support and resources, consider blended courses and build support for an online program for future courses. A blended course combines technology and traditional classroom strategies. Developing a blended course is an excellent strategy to begin while gathering resources, support, and experience. Gravitate toward a level at which the effort will be successful. Maximize the resources available and incorporate new resources and technology that will enhance the courses. Pilot the material, have the material peer reviewed, and solicit learner feedback frequently for incorporation into course revisions.

RECONCEPTUALIZING A COURSE

An undergraduate Community/Public Health Nursing course was transferred to the online environment. The content outline was developed as follows:

Community/Public Health Nursing
Module 1: History of Community/Public Health Nursing
Objectives and Readings
Content
Activities

Module 2: Influences on the Practice of Community/Public Health Nursing
Objectives and Readings
Content
Activities

History and scope	Focus
Practice	Tools

FIGURE 6.2 The reconceptualized course.

Module 3: Cultural Influences on the Practice of Community/Public Health Nursing
Objectives and Readings
Content
Activities

This organizing framework continued to Module 15 for a 15-week course. This design was cumbersome and needed streamlining. Upon examining the content, the course really contained four areas of content: History and Scope, Practice, Focus, and Tools. The modules were shifted into four content areas as illustrated in Figure 6.2.

Each content area contains several of the original modules. History and Scope comprises Modules 1, 2, and 3; Practice comprises Modules 4, 5, 6, and 7; Focus comprises Modules 8 and 9; and Tools comprises Modules 10, 11, and 12. The content areas and the modules within that area are color coded in the same color. Each module contains objectives and readings, minilectures, podcasts, and activities. This reconceptualization has several advantages. Students repeatedly see the four content areas, and these become the four concepts of Community/Public Health Nursing. The concepts, called *mental models*, provide consistent reinforcement each time the student accesses the course content. Mental models give meaning to concepts and promote the transfer of knowledge from the "didactic" to the "real" world. When the student repeatedly sees the word *Tools*, the student forms a mental model that community/public health nursing has tools, and one of those tools is epidemiology (a module). Operationalizing the mental model in an activity strengthens its impact. For example, one of the activities in the Tools could include a case study of an epidemic of influenza in a community. Reconceptualizing a course provides students with a "map" of the course so they can see what the course is about, where they have been, and where they are going in the course.

SUMMARY

Decisions about moving a course or program online can be guided by using a decision tree. Examples of decisions include whether a course should be taught in a blended learning environment or totally online. The stage between making the decision to use online learning strategies and actually developing the learning environment is most important. Reconceptualizing the learning environment means going from, "Okay, I have this learning material," to using online pedagogy, infrastructure, and technology to make decisions about how the learning material will be presented online. Reconceptualizing a program is using a series of "if–then" statements to make decisions. It is a decision tree in which strengths, purposes, and resources are examined to make decisions concerning the best approach to use in presenting the learning material. Reconceptualizing is answering questions and using the answers to guide the development of online learning environments. The decision tree will then guide your decision-making. It comprises questions, possible answers, and possible actions. Questions are posed about institutional issues, technology, faculty, and students. Possible answers to the questions are given, and actions based on each of the possible responses are proposed. Reconceptualizing a course is characterized by forming mental models that guide the decisions about the course, such as how the modules will be organized, and what will be the format of the modules. The modules will include objectives, content, teaching strategies, and evaluation.

7

Practical Applications in Academic Online Learning Environments

Kathleen M. Buckley

INTRODUCTION

The term *blended learning* is often used interchangeably with other terms in educational and research realms. Blended learning is also referred to as hybrid learning, mixed mode learning, web-enhanced instruction, technology-enhanced instruction, and technology-mediated instruction. In recent years, *blended learning* has been used with more regularity and is becoming the accepted term for education that combines face-to-face instruction with computer-mediated activities. Allen and Seaman (2016) define blended courses and programs as having between 30% and 80% of content delivered online (technology mediated) and the remainder delivered in a traditional, face-to-face environment. Technology-mediated instruction occurs with users in different physical locations, and the face-to-face instruction occurs with them in the same physical space.

Blended learning has been described by educators and students as combining the best elements of traditional and online learning (Adams Becker et al., 2017). In a national survey of 232 faculty members teaching in higher education about their use of technology, 73% of the respondents reported blended learning as being the most common model in use (Kelly, 2017). In another national survey of chief academic officers, blended-learning outcomes were reported to be the same as (56.6%) or superior to (35.6%) those in face-to-face instruction (Allen & Seaman, 2016). This finding is consistent with that of at least two meta-analyses in which students in blended courses were found to perform consistently better than those with traditional face-to-face instruction (Means, Toyama, Murphy, & Baki, 2013; Vo, Zhua, & Diepa, 2017).

The blended-learning approach can occur at the course level, the program level, or the institutional level (Drysdale, Graham, Spring, & Halverson, 2013; Porter, Graham, Spring, & Welch, 2014; Vaughan & Cloutier, 2016). At the course level, the blending of delivery modes occurs for a single subject over the span of one semester. At the program level, the blended approach ensues across courses in a program; selected courses may be completely online while others are taught in a traditional face-to-face format. At an institutional level, the blended model can be expanded so that an institution uses the combined approach to deliver all of its course offerings. The last approach is used by many of the state virtual school supplemental online programs.

ORGANIZING THE DELIVERY AND CONTENT

Blended learning is not traditional face-to-face instruction, and it is not online learning; it is its own instructional strategy and therefore needs to be approached differently than other formats. The delivery format and repertoire of learning tools need to be addressed when going through the process of designing a course. This is especially true when approaching blended learning. Blended learning has the opportunity to take on endless forms, so the relationship between content and delivery needs to be carefully planned. It would be a disservice to students, faculty, and the institution for a traditionally classroom-based course or a fully online course to use the same educational approaches and content in a blended-learning approach.

DELIVERY FORMATS

A variety of delivery formats are becoming available for blended learning. The most common include face-to-face, in-class sessions on campus coupled with online activities. Flipped classrooms that employ both online and face-to-face classes are growing in popularity as a blended format. In a national survey, 61% of faculty stated that at least one of their classes was flipped (Kelly, 2017). In many programs, web conferencing is also becoming a part of the blended format, where by students meet face to face via cameras and microphones to interact in real time from a distance coupled with online modules.

CLASSROOM-BASED SESSIONS

When deciding how best to use classroom-based sessions, faculty may consider their use as excellent opportunities for community building. Kear, Chetwynd, and Jefferis (2014) regard social presence as a critical element in community building. Social presence theory, developed by Short, Williams, and Christie (1976), has been defined as the degree to which people are perceived as being real persons rather than objects. It is reinforced by communicating with other participants in a course not only through physical indicators such as eye contact, body language, and a projection of interest or excitement, but also through exchanges of information via dialogue. Holding some classes face to face in a classroom allows an instructor to take maximum advantage of this type of communication among students to reinforce social presence and bonding. However, spending the session lecturing on a particular topic or focusing on the mechanics of a course management system does little to reinforce establishing a relationship among faculty and students, and minimizes the opportunity for community building. Activities should be carefully planned to reinforce and encourage social presence.

Introductions are an easy way to reinforce social presence in the first session. This activity gives faculty and students the ability to closely view physical characteristics, such as mannerisms, gestures, voice tone and quality, and all that goes into making them unique persons, while taking in the information that they are sharing about themselves. Introductions might be followed by learning activities that encourage students not only to interact, but also to create opportunities for sharing and collaborative learning.

Being able to manipulate the physical environment easily is another advantage of on-campus or virtual, face-to-face meetings. Small-group work is relatively easy in this kind of setting. Students can be asked to quickly rearrange themselves in groups and discuss a series of questions on the content, work on a case study, or review and critique evidence-based articles. Engagement through these kinds of active learning activities is the first step toward building a sense of comfort and security among students, which helps them to achieve self-confidence, a necessary component of collaboration. Interaction in the classroom has been reported as being more in-depth than that in the online learning mode (Shu & Gu, 2018).

Many programs schedule the last class as a face-to-face, on-campus session. This time is often used for student presentations as a means to evaluate their understanding of the content. However, viewing multiple, back-to-back student presentations can quickly lead to audience burnout with little learning occurring. With the availability of recording capabilities through web conferencing, presentations can now be recorded by students and posted for viewing asynchronously by the instructor and their peers. A final class session can then be used for more in-depth discussion of the presentations that have already been viewed. With the current ease in recording, there is no longer any need to use classroom time for watching presentations. It may be of greater value to schedule an in-class session earlier in the term and use it for activities that are best accomplished face to face.

ONLINE DELIVERY

The online delivery format allows for a multitude of other learning activities, depending on the features of the available course management system. Faculty should carefully prepare to take advantage of any available instructional technologies that may encourage interaction among students and continue to build the community of learning. These interactive activities may include discussion board questions, wikis, blogs, or the posting of voice/video threads (Adelman & Nogueras, 2013). Because there is a greater risk of students experiencing feelings of isolation in the online environment, technology that supports social presence helps learners feel a more personal and emotional connection as part of a community. For example, community building can continue with online introductions on a discussion board, which offers the advantage of being readily available for those who wish to refresh their memory of a faculty member's or student's background. One of the best uses of the online format is in providing text or lectures in the format of slides or videos that present new information. In flipped classrooms, online instruction often through recorded lectures or readings is used to prepare the students for the classroom face-to-face sessions.

WEB CONFERENCING

Web conferencing is another format that offers another dimension of being able to interact "face to face" as in a classroom but via the Internet and the use of audio–video technology. With classroom-based discussion, there is the advantage of giving and receiving immediate feedback, which may create an illusion in which the technology almost disappears and participants have the sense of being together in the same place. The best use of this delivery format is again not with a lecture—lectures can be videotaped and placed in online modules for convenient and repeated viewing. The opportunity for interaction should be optimized with group activities and discussions.

One superior advantage of web conferencing is being able to bring guest experts who are at a distance to the sessions. In a classroom-based course, because of the expense and inconvenience, it may be impossible for students to meet with these experts, but with web conferencing, the only things needed are the expert's willingness, time for the session itself, and access to a camera, microphone, and the Internet. Some web-conferencing systems even allow for break-out rooms in which students can meet separately in smaller groups and then come back to the entire class and share the highlights of their group work. Student presentations are also an activity that may be maximized via web conferencing, although if the classes are large, it may be better to have the students record their presentations and post them for viewing prior to the web-conferencing session. In that way, the time together as a class can be used to discuss and critique what has already been viewed.

SCHEDULING OF DELIVERY FORMATS

Most blended programs have a preset schedule of delivery formats to coordinate students coming to campus for several courses during the same period of time. For example, students may be scheduled to attend in-class sessions the first and last weeks of the semester, with online course work and periodic web-conferencing sessions making up the balance of course delivery formats over the rest of the semester. Schedules are usually developed and circulated to the students prior to the start of the semester, so that they are able to plan their professional and personal responsibilities around class meetings on campus or via web conferencing. Other courses are designed around the flipped classroom, in which students are asked to view recorded lectures in advance of a face-to-face class, in which more active learning strategies are used.

Fitting the content of a course within a preset schedule of delivery format may require some adjustment in the organization of course content.

MAXIMIZING THE SCHEDULE

In a classroom-based course, the content may usually be covered in a set order, such as one that may mimic the order of the chapters in the accompanying textbook. However, it is not always possible for the content to be covered in its natural order, as the schedule for the different modes of delivery may be set by the school or program. These schedules are often driven by days and times most convenient to the student population to be able to attend face-to-face or online synchronous sessions, distance-learning students who may have to travel to attend on-campus classes, availability of meeting spaces, and the need for technical or specialized support. For example, personnel may be available only on certain days and times to cover instructional activities in a clinical simulation environment, or online activities may need to be scheduled around known downtime for the online technology platform.

If the schedule is preset for a blended course, instructors should consider how to best match the content and approaches with delivery format. This can be done by mapping the delivery formats against module objectives, content to be covered, instructional strategies, and methods of assessment and evaluation. See Table 7.1 for an example of mapping for a Nursing Informatics course consisting of online learning combined with in-class and web-conferencing sessions. The faculty should place a high priority on maintaining curricular integrity and quality during this planning process to ensure that content delivered via web-based formats meets the same academic standard of excellence as the face-to-face format. Following the same order in the blended format may underutilize the available course delivery mode. Attention should be given to ensure that the delivery format is being used to its best advantage. The best case is when the content drives the delivery format, as this allows for the greatest use of available resources.

CLARIFYING THE BLENDED FORMAT FOR STUDENTS

Although it may be apparent to faculty why a course is considered "blended," it cannot be assumed that students will have a clear understanding. It should be explicitly stated at the start of the course in a "welcome" announcement that the course is blended and what delivery formats will be used. The purpose of the different delivery formats

TABLE 7.1 Mapping of Course Delivery Format

Course Delivery Format	Module Objectives	Content	Activities	Evaluation
In-class session	Module 1: Information Theories and Models • Discern the relevance of informatics to DNP practice • Analyze the data, information, knowledge, and wisdom (D–I–K–W) model and other theories used in informatics practice • Evaluate the relevance of the D–I–K–W model in healthcare technology and student's specific area of interest	Nursing science and its relationship to nursing roles and nursing informatics Introduction to D–I–K–W model Transforming nursing practice through technology	Required readings Class discussion	In-class participation and verbal feedback from peers and faculty
Online session	Module 2: The Model: Data, Information, Knowledge, Wisdom? • Evaluate how information technology impacts nursing practice • Assess how information technologies impact the role of nurses as knowledge workers • Develop recommendations to improve the system for use by nurses	Overview of nursing informatics How health information technologies impact nursing practice	Readings Discussion board question	Discussion board participation rubric

(continued)

TABLE 7.1   **Mapping of Course Delivery Format** *(continued)*

Course Delivery Format	Module Objectives	Content	Activities	Evaluation
Online session	Module 3: Information Science—The Foundation of Knowledge • Categorize the types of knowledge provided by a real-world information system or technology • Decide how that knowledge may generate practice wisdom • Describe how data from one information system create information that generates knowledge, which builds wisdom and influences nursing practice	How information systems generate knowledge that influences nursing practice	Required readings Student group work via web conferencing outside of class meetings with posting of group response on course discussion board	Group assignment rubric
Web-conferencing session	Module 4: Selecting and Evaluating an Information System • Identify the Systems Development Life Cycle (found in the course material) as the best practice process for system implementation • Support the value of the DNP role in the life cycle process • Construct a potential plan for evaluation of the system	Selection and evaluation of an information system The Systems Development Life Cycle and the nursing role	Required readings Interview of user engaged in implementation of health care information system Sharing of interview results and discussion via web-conferencing class	Participation in web-conferencing group discussion and verbal feedback from peers and faculty

DNP, Doctor of Nursing Practice.

should be explained to students to help them understand how and why these formats are important to the learning process. A general statement might be used in the welcome statement, such as "The blended format is designed to give students the opportunity to combine the convenience of online coursework with more real-time, individualized attention that meets a variety of learning styles. In-class and web-conferencing sessions allow students to participate in face-to-face interactive contact with instructors and peers." Students will also need to know where to find the delivery components of the course, when and where they should participate each week, and a structured set of topics and schedule for each specifying the dates, times, and locations of synchronous meetings.

Clarification of course delivery methods might be made by creating separate modules for in-class, online, and web-conferencing sessions. Then, in the introduction to each module, the course delivery format could be highlighted with a rationale as to why that particular format is being used to cover selected content. Separate modules for in-class and web-conferencing sessions might also be included, with specific objectives for those sessions as well as directions on how to prepare for the sessions with requirements for participation. For other courses that may have online and clinical delivery components, modules may be used to cover the information to be delivered online, and a separate section created in the course management system detailing the information and schedule related to the clinical aspect of the course.

CONNECTING LEARNING ACTIVITIES ACROSS DELIVERY FORMATS

Although the delivery format for particular learning activities should be clear to the students, the connections among them across formats should also be obvious. For example, faculty might initially assign readings, short videos, or taped lectures as an introduction to content, and make these available to students asynchronously online. These kinds of activities might be followed by a face-to-face classroom-based or web-conferencing session with the purpose of having the students engage in a discussion of the material they previously reviewed with a set of structured questions. Sequencing these activities within the same learning module on a specific theme clarifies the relationship between the activities, and acknowledges their mutual reinforcement of each other.

Another example of connecting activities across delivery formats occurs with faculty and student introductions. If the course begins with a classroom-based session, introductions of faculty and students can easily be incorporated into the class activities. Introductions serve a number of purposes. They are the first step in developing relationships among the faculty and students to build a community of learning, and they create a sense of connection. Faculty introductions also are an opportunity to share one's background and expertise, philosophy of learning, role in the course, and experience in teaching blended courses. The introduction should also be delivered in a manner that encourages approachability.

Even if introductions are begun in a live interactive session, best practices support repeating them online in blended courses. This repetition not only serves as a reminder to students who may have forgotten what was said during the initial session, but also is available to students who may have missed the session. The online introduction may include all that was shared in the real-time session as well as a picture, email address, phone number, and best days and times to be reached by phone or email. With the increase in diversity of cultures of students, the introduction should include the instructor's preference on how he or she wishes to be addressed. It is up to the faculty member whether to also include personal information such as family and interests outside his or her professional life. However, many instructors feel that sharing some personal information increases the sense of social presence, or helps them to be seen as real persons rather than objects, and contributes toward becoming more approachable by students.

Student introductions are also extremely helpful in building the learning community and making those connections. Students can learn much from their peers if they are comfortable to interact with them. Again, even if students have an opportunity to introduce themselves during an initial live session, it should also be available online for future reference. Clear instructions on what to include in the introduction should be given, and students should be encouraged to share some personal information. It is often this kind of information that helps other students gravitate toward someone who shares their same background or interests and helps them begin to build a personal connection.

ADVANTAGES AND DISADVANTAGES OF BLENDED LEARNING

The number one advantage of the blended approach is that it empowers the faculty and the student to utilize all available avenues for both teaching and learning. The delivery of the teaching can take on many different formats and use multiple technologies to achieve a single objective. Okaz (2015) summarizes the advantages of blended learning for both faculty and students: easier access to information, convenience, thoughtful participation, ability to use electronic tools and the Internet, independent learning, and better learning outcomes. Instructors have the flexibility to choose an instructional method and modality that best fits their teaching style, the content to be covered, and the targeted objective. This same flexibility transfers to students. Students with different learning styles are given the opportunity to gravitate toward the methods that best reach them. These opportunities can be seen in the chosen delivery of the content, the flexibility of when and where to consume the content, and the possibilities of how to complete an assignment.

It is noteworthy that student satisfaction and performance have been reported to be improved with blended learning, and an environment that permits student–teacher–content interaction (Bernard, Borokhovski, Schmid, & Abrami, 2014; Ma'arop & Embi, 2016; Vo et al., 2017). In particular, flipped classrooms have been associated with higher learning outcomes when compared with traditional lecture-based learning (Chen et al., 2018). However, there is also debate as to whether the effect is primarily due to the use of active learning strategies in the classroom (Jensen, Kummer, & de Melo Godoy, 2015). It could be that the same findings would have occurred through the use of active learning strategies in a fully online course, such as discussion boards, wikis, blogs, online exercises, small group projects, group problem-solving assignments, or peer critiques.

Although most traditional face-to-face courses are able to meet the needs of students who fall within the middle of the bell curve in relation to meeting the learning objectives of the course, some students need a different approach to be successful. A blended-learning approach allows the instructor to offer more occasions for students who may need remediation to be successful in gaining a deeper understanding of content. It may also provide more flexibility in offering opportunities for students to pursue their interests well beyond the required objectives of the course. This flexibility also gives seasoned students more opportunities in a variety of formats to be successful and get the most out of their educational experience.

Although the flexibility available through a blended-learning approach may be seen as a significant advantage, it can also become a disadvantage in that the complexity of learning modes can be overwhelming for some faculty and students. If a faculty member or student has not previously experienced a blended course or program, it may be difficult to grasp the individual components and how they fit together. The core components of good course design need to be applied to and emphasized with the blended model, as they are sometimes overshadowed by the sheer complexity of the design. It is also important for both groups to have a strong orientation to the blended approach including how it relates to their role. The orientation should start with the whole picture view to ensure understanding of the entire system, and then focus on the components of the system.

There can also be a lack of flexibility if the instructor has to quickly move content from one format to another. Because so much planning goes into having the different delivery modes "fit" together, when an event requires an immediate change in delivery format, the process can have a snowball effect. For example, a face-to-face, classroom-based session may have to be abruptly canceled because of bad weather, or a technical problem may cause a web-conferencing session to crash. Because these delivery modes were most likely selected as the best format for meeting specific learning objectives or delivering particular exercises and activities, having to accommodate a last-minute change can be formidable. Often, synchronous sessions are planned months in advance with guest speakers and prescheduled space. Rescheduling the session may be highly problematic or impossible. At the last minute, the instructor may have to revise the entire lesson plan into an asynchronous format.

Another disadvantage relates to the technical context within which the student and faculty are consuming the technology-delivered material. Although most academic settings post minimum technical specifications on admission and all content should be created with those specifications in mind, access to the Internet is not always a known variable or a controllable one. The ways in which students experience e-learning techniques are strongly influenced by Internet connectivity and broadband levels.

Blended courses can provide both new opportunities and advantages for students with learning disabilities, but at the same time, they bring the difficulties of the classroom and online environment with them (Heiman, Fichten, Olenik-Shemesh, Keshet, & Jorgensen, 2017; Rivera, 2017). For example, the online mode of delivery may be more convenient and accessible for students with mobility impairments. In contrast, students with learning disabilities or other less visible disabilities may be less likely to self-disclose their disability and seek accommodations.

FACULTY AND COURSE EVALUATIONS IN A BLENDED COURSE

A strong evaluation plan is essential for faculty to improve their courses, as well as enhance and ensure quality education for students. The evaluation strategies should be designed to elicit feedback on all aspects of the blended course. The purpose is to obtain student perceptions about the instructional strategies, learning activities/resources, technological aspects of the course, and course delivery formats. However, the evaluation strategies for a blended course should be less focused on the technology and mode of course delivery, and should explore the effectiveness of the delivery format for achieving the learning objectives. For example, a 5-point Likert scale ranging from Strongly Disagree to Strongly Agree might be used for evaluation purposes, and it includes the following statements:

- The amount of contact with the instructor has met my needs.
- The balance of course delivery formats facilitated meeting the course objectives.
- Working on group assignments with my peers via web conferencing has contributed to a sense of a learning community.

Periodic assessments can be scheduled during the in-class and web-conferencing sessions in which discussions or interactive exercises may serve as opportunities for a formative evaluation of students' understanding of the content presented online. Mid-semester evaluations can be very useful in identifying strengths and weaknesses in the course, which can allow for immediate improvements to the course. End-of-course summative evaluations of blended courses offer students a means to provide input for assessing and improving course design, course delivery, and teaching performance. Through anonymous end-of-semester course evaluations, students give instructors and the university feedback about the effectiveness, quality, and value of courses. This feedback often plays an important role in course improvement as well as faculty review processes.

Faculty teaching blended courses benefit from using established benchmarks when designing and evaluating their courses. The Quality

Matters program has received national recognition for developing a research-based rubric consisting of eight general standards and 42 specific criteria that describe best practices in online and blended learning. The rubric is used as part of a collaborative peer review process with the primary aim of ensuring quality assurance and continuous improvement. The rubric includes annotations that are focused specifically on blended courses, and provides recommendations for how to handle introductions, scheduling, explanations of purposes of delivery formats, and connections/sequencing among the course delivery modes. Other similar tools are available for the design and evaluation of blended courses, such as the OLC (Online Learning Consortium) Quality Scorecard for Blended-Learning Programs. Institutions can use this scorecard to identify strengths and weaknesses within their courses or programs, and develop a strategy for meeting the benchmarks.

SUMMARY

Blended-learning courses and programs offer the majority of content delivered online with the remainder delivered in a traditional, face-to-face environment. Blended learning has been described by educators and students as combining the best elements of traditional and online learning. In this chapter, a variety of delivery formats that have been used for blended learning are described, highlighting the advantages and challenges of each. Also discussed are considerations in scheduling the various delivery formats as well as the importance of clarifying for the students why a course is being delivered in a blended format. The chapter ends with emphasis on the importance of a strong formative and summative evaluation plan for blended courses.

REFERENCES

Adams Becker, S., Cummins, M., Davis, A., Freeman, A., Hall Giesinger, C., & Ananthanarayanan, V. (2017). *NMC horizon report: 2017 higher education edition.* Austin, TX: The New Media Consortium.

Adelman, D. S., & Nogueras, D. J. (2013). Discussion boards: Boring no more! *Nurse Educator, 38*(1), 30–33. doi:10.1097/NNE.0b013e318276df77

Allen, L. A., & Seaman, J. (2016). *Online report card: Tracking education in the United States.* Retrieved from https://www.onlinelearningsurvey.com/reports/Online ReportCard_embargo.pdf

Bernard, R. M., Borokhovski, E., Schmid, R. F., & Abrami, P. C. (2014). A meta-analysis of blended learning and technology use in higher education: From the general to the applied. *Journal of Computing in Higher Education, 26*(1), 87–122. doi:10.1007/s12528-013-9077-3

Chen, K. S., Monrouxe, L., Lu, Y. H., Jeng, C. C., Chang, Y. J., & Chai, P. Y. C. (2018). Academic outcomes of flipped classroom learning: A meta-analysis. *Medical Education in Review, 52,* 910–924. doi:10.1111/medu.13616

Drysdale, J. S., Graham, C. R., Spring, K. J., & Halverson, L. R. (2013). An analysis of research trends in dissertations and theses studying blended learning. *Internet and Higher Education, 17,* 90–100. doi:10.1016/j.iheduc.2012.11.003

Heiman, T., Fichten, C. S., Olenik-Shemesh, D., Keshet, N. S., & Jorgensen, M. (2017). Access and perceived ICT usability among students with disabilities attending higher education institutions. *Education and Information Technologies, 22*(6), 2727–2740. doi:10.1007/s10639-017-9623-0

Jensen, J. L., Kummer, T. A., & de Melo Godoy, P. D. (2015). Improvements from a flipped classroom may simply be the fruits of active learning. *CBE Life Sciences Education, 13*(1), ar 5. doi:10.1187/cbe.14-08-0129

Kear, K., Chetwynd, F., & Jefferis, H. (2014). Social presence in online learning communities: The role of personal profile. *Research in Learning Technology, 22,* 19710. doi:10.3402/rlt.v22.19710

Kelly, R. (2017). 2017 teaching with technology survey. *Campus Technology, 30*(7), 25–37. Retrieved from https://digital.1105media.com/CampusTech/2017/CAM_1707/SY_1707Q1_701925010.html#p=25

Ma'arop, A. H., & Embi, M. A. (2016). Implementation of blended learning in higher learning institutions: A review of the literature. *International Education Studies, 9*(3), 41–52. doi:10.5539/ies.v9n3p41

Means, B., Toyama, Y., Murphy, R., & Baki, M. (2013). The effectiveness of online and blended learning: A meta-analysis of the empirical literature. *Teachers College Record, 115,* 030303. Retrieved from https://www.sri.com/sites/default/files/publications/effectiveness_of_online_and_blended_learning.pdf

Okaz, A. A. (2015). Integrating blended learning in higher education. *Procedia – Social and Behavioral Sciences, 186*(2015), 600–603. doi:10.1016/j.sbspro.2015.04.086

Porter, W. W., Graham, C. R., Spring, K. A., & Welch, K. R. (2014). Blended learning in higher education: Institutional adoption and implementation. *Computers & Education, 75*(2014), 185–195. doi:10.1016/j.compedu.2014.02.011

Rivera, J. H. (2017). The blended learning environment: A viable alternative for special needs students. *Journal of Education and Training Studies, 5*(2), 79–84. doi:10.11114/jets.v5i2.2125

Short, J., Williams, E., & Christie, B. (1976). *The social psychology of telecommunications.* London, England: John Wiley & Sons.

Shu, H., & Gu, X. (2018). Determining the differences between online and face-to-face student–group interactions in a blended learning course. *The Internet and Higher Education, 39,* 13–21. doi:10.1016/j.iheduc.2018.05.003

Vaughan, N. D., & Cloutier, D. (2016). A programmatic approach to blended learning. In A. Volungeviciene, A. Szűcs, & I. Mázár (Eds.), *9th EDEN Research Workshop: Forging new pathways of research and innovation in open and distance learning* (pp. 200–211). Budapest, Hungary: European Distance and E-Learning Network. Retrieved from http://www.eden-online.org/wp-content/uploads/2016/10/RW_2016_Oldenburg_Proceedings.pdf

Vo, M. H., Zhua, C., & Diepa, N. A. (2017). The effect of blended learning on student performance at course-level in higher education: A meta-analysis. *Studies in Educational Evaluation, 53,* 17–28. doi:10.1016/j.stueduc.2017.01.002

Practical Applications in Professional Online Learning Environments

Susan L. Bindon

INTRODUCTION

Nurses and clinical staff who work in hospitals and many other professional settings need continuous education and updates to maintain their competence (Bindon, 2017). Newly hired staff are typically oriented to the organization, the department, and their specific role in the workplace. Clinicians in these settings must stay abreast of the latest evidence and apply it to their practice. To do so, they need to be informed of regulatory changes, practice guidelines, policy and procedure revisions, and equipment updates. They may seek education or training on nonclinical aspects of their role, such as communication or leadership skills. Clinicians are also obligated to maintain competence with relevant technical skills and often require education and targeted practice to do so. Patients and their families expect competence and high-quality, error-free care from providers. In many respects, learning and professional development are part of daily life for clinicians. Hospital or site-based education quite literally picks up where academic or professional education leaves off and continues throughout one's career. Lifelong learning is a key component of safe, competent nursing practice. This chapter explores application of online learning in the professional practice environment, the impact on both learners and educators, and the outcomes that can be supported or realized by its use. Various workplace elements make the use of online learning in the practice setting a unique challenge.

BACKGROUND

The American Nurses Association's (ANA) position paper on professional role competence states that nurses and employers share responsibility for professional competence (ANA, 2014). The individual nurse is accountable for his or her own practice, and employers are responsible for creating an environment conducive to safe, competent care. The ANA further extends accountability to include the profession, professional organizations, credentialing and certification entities, regulatory agencies, and other key stakeholders. Nursing professional development (NPD) practitioners—a title adopted by the Association for Nursing Professional Development (Harper & Maloney, 2016)—play a key part in this arena and are largely responsible for initial and ongoing education of clinical staff across specialties and disciplines. These nurse educators use knowledge and skills in education theory, design, career development, leadership, and program management to "influence professional role competence and professional growth of learners in a variety of settings and support lifelong learners in an interprofessional environment that facilitates continuous development and learning" (Harper & Maloney, 2016, p. 63). These varied responsibilities and their scope of practice require NPD practitioners to work creatively, efficiently, and at a high competence level in overlapping professional contexts—clinical practice and education. At the same time, they must have working knowledge of complex systems, quality improvement and implementation science, informatics, and return on investment from a financial perspective. These skills are reflected in the seven subroles (learning facilitator, change agent, mentor, leader, champion for scientific inquiry, advocate for NPD specialty, and partner for practice transitions) identified in the NPD Practice Model, a simple yet comprehensive input–throughput–output model. The model is depicted and described more fully by Rheingans (2016).

As learning facilitators, NPD practitioners have expertise in applying the education process to address learning needs. The education process closely resembles the six-step nursing process and helps to guide one's work. First, NPD educators *assess* learning needs and identify baseline knowledge and skill levels. Needs assessments are done using survey, observation, interview, pretest, or learner self-assessment data. Online surveys sent via an organization's secure email system using survey software such as SurveyMonkey or Qualtrics are commonly used to collect assessment and evaluation data before and after an education program. Educators then *validate* their assessment with stakeholders to *identify outcomes* that are realistic and attainable within the organizational culture and context. At this stage, *planning* begins. Educators write learner-centered objectives and design content. They select teaching and evaluation strategies that support the objectives and desired outcomes. NPD educators then *implement* the education plan, and finally they *evaluate* learners' achievement of objectives and the effectiveness of the overall plan. Lesson or program plans are useful to align objectives, content, projected outcomes, teaching strategies, technology needs, learning and evaluation activities, time frames, and necessary resources. These plans also help to ensure consistency among presenters, document NPD responses to learning needs, and provide a template for design of future versions of the class or course. Program plans can be developed and shared electronically and are easily retrievable for The Joint Commission, Magnet®, Centers for Medicare and Medicaid Services, board of nursing, continuing education (CE), or other regulatory queries and purposes.

To briefly illustrate this process and to know how it might be used, consider the following scenario. Based on latest evidence and standards of care, an organization decides to implement a new patient identification process, moving from bar code technology to biometric patient identification (e.g., palm scans, digital fingerprints, and facial recognition). NPD is asked to educate staff about the new process in time for go-live, just 2 months away. Using their needs assessment skills, educators might determine that all clinical staff (1,000+ learners) require education. Content will focus on the need for the identification methods, the intended outcome of the new technologies, current patient identification policy, staff's responsibility when identifying patients, the use of new equipment, and resources for troubleshooting. The educators share this assessment with key stakeholders who agree to the scope, objectives, and target outcomes. Next, the educators decide to use a blended learning approach to this project. They design an online module including rationale for the change (inconsistent patient identification and rising error rates), the current policy, a video demonstrating scanner use, links to external resources and evidence on biometrics for patient safety, and a short self-assessment or quiz. They pilot the module with representative learners and determine the learning level is appropriate for all identified users. Educators also schedule multiple drop-in sessions in upcoming weeks to demonstrate the use of the scanner and allow learners to practice. The online module is assigned to all clinical staff by job title and code, communication is extended to learners regarding access and availability, and the module is launched. Course completion is tracked via the organization's learning management system (LMS), and weekly electronic progress reports are generated for stakeholders. Educators also plan to provide at-the-elbow support on the units for 1 week after go-live to answer questions and to ensure adoption. They then evaluate the efficiency and effectiveness of the plan using module completion data, unit observations, and incident report data on patient identification for the next quarter. In this scenario, using a blended format and online learning module allowed NPD educators to deliver a consistent high-stakes message to a wide audience in a relatively short time. Learners unable to complete the education during the allotted time due to illness, vacation, or family leave time can complete the online module upon their return.

In addition to their role as educators, NPD practitioners act as change agents for unit-based or system-wide projects, are recognized leaders within an organization, and promote the translation of evidence into practice. They are subject-matter experts (SMEs) on a wide range of clinical, technological, and regulatory topics. Sometimes these nurses act as facilitators of the education process rather than the actual presenters or instructors, supporting the notion that the clinical workplace requires NPD educators to be learning experts. In short, the role of NPD specialists is broad and constantly evolves to meet the demands of the organization and the learners to whom they are accountable. As far back as 2004, Shanley stated the staff educator's role includes facilitating staff adoption of technology. Since then, the role has expanded to include the design, use, and evaluation of online learning and web-based education strategies.

Emphasis on the use of technology to facilitate learning, such as simulation, distance, and web-based learning, was identified as an emerging trend for the NPD specialty in their Scope and Standards of Practice (Harper & Maloney, 2016). NPD practitioners need to be flexible and future focused in response to emerging trends in practice and education. Use of smartphones, watches, and other mobile devices by patients, staff, and educators; the explosion of social media; virtual learning environments; telehealth options; and cyber vulnerabilities were listed among those to watch (Harper & Maloney, 2016). According to one survey, 65% of nurses use a mobile device onsite for professional purposes, 20% for 2 hours or more per day, and most of them use mobile apps to locate information in the clinical setting (Wolters Kluwer Health, 2014). With nurses turning to mobile technology to access clinical information, it is imperative that the content is accurate and trustworthy. Organizations need to decide what information employees can access and how they can do so. NPD practitioners need to lead change in how we teach and learn in the workplace.

LEARNERS

In contrast to an academic setting where students in a particular class have relatively similar goals and ability levels, a unique challenge for NPD specialists is the variety of learners for which they may be responsible. Though often questioned, there is no definitive "right size" span of control or ratio of learners to educators in NPD. Depending on the topic, learners can include interprofessional team members (nurses, physicians, therapists), unlicensed workers (technicians, support staff, environmental services), nonclinical staff (security, transportation, admitting personnel), and students from many disciplines. Inherent among these learners is a wide range of learning styles, ages, cultural backgrounds, literacy levels, languages, and other learning preferences and abilities. Added to this is the challenge of reaching learners in a 24-7 environment where they may work irregular schedules and shifts. There is little time for clinical staff to be away from patient care responsibilities to attend classes or take advantage of optional educational offerings.

Learners in a clinical setting are by and large adult employees, students, or volunteers. They are busy, flexible, and mobile, and educators must be ready to respond to not only their learning needs but also their learning expectations. Expectations can vary greatly as multiple generations come together in the workplace. For example, in contrast to traditional learners accustomed to face-to-face or assigned online learning experiences, Generation Z learners (born roughly between 1995 and 2012) entering the workplace may expect learning that is individualized, on demand, engaging, visual, and technology based or accessible (Chicca & Shellenbarger, 2018). Educators also need to consider learner motivations. Unlike students in an academic setting, employees are not concerned with grades and progression through a program of study. Motivators for these learners may include reaching internal goals such as gaining a certification in a nursing specialty or becoming a preceptor; external motivators may include increased salary or expanded job opportunities.

In some instances, employees engage in learning following a mandate from supervisors or the organization itself and are largely motivated by a need to be "signed off." These requirements, particularly related to electronic health record education, have been identified as a contributing factor to physician and caregiver burnout (Valentine, 2018). Determining the best way to engage diverse, distracted, and often stressed adults to complete mandatory training or elective courses presents a significant challenge for NPD specialists. Online learning approaches can help by adding convenient and flexible options to NPD instructors' repertoire of teaching strategies.

EDUCATORS

Education in hospital and academic settings differs in several ways. NPD educators are usually outstanding clinicians who have an interest in education design and delivery and may be certified as NPD educators. Some have advanced degrees with an education focus; others have no formal background in education. Currently, there are two recognized levels of NPD practitioners: the NPD generalist (a bachelor's prepared nurse with or without NPD certification or a master's prepared nurse without certification) and an NPD specialist (a master's prepared nurse certified in NPD; Harper & Maloney, 2016). Of note, *technology* is one of the categories on the NPD certification exam, making up 7% of the total questions (American Nurses Credentialing Center, 2018). Subtopics cover information management and technology tools, including online learning.

NPD educators are typically responsible for addressing staff learning needs across defined areas. One educator may cover several nursing units within a service line (acute care, rehabilitation, perioperative), rather than teaching a specific number of courses or credits within a defined program. NPD educators design annual education schedules, but in contrast to academia, hospital-based education has no firm academic calendar. Timelines develop as needs arise throughout the year. Within this framework, NPD educators must adjust and reprioritize as needed to address issues of patient safety, risk management, and occasional unexpected events. It is nearly impossible to plan ahead for unforeseen events requiring just-in-time (JIT) training. It is equally difficult to develop and deliver a quality product given a short turnaround time. Learners have a similarly hard time absorbing and making sense of information when bombarded from several angles at once. Wright (2005) suggests that to function in such a pressured environment, every nurse needs the ability to "learn on the fly." Finding needed resources and quickly learning the essentials when faced with the new or unfamiliar is the hallmark of this type of teaching and learning. It is critical to understand that online learning in this environment demands a change in practice not only for learners but also for NPD educators. They become more facilitative and less instructive, more guiding and less authoritative (Gormley, 2013).

ENVIRONMENTS/SETTINGS

Depending on the size of the organization, education departments' range can be from one NPD generalist in a rural setting to dozens of highly specialized educators across a multisite system. How departments are organized (centralized or decentralized) and whether or not education is viewed as a value-added investment largely depend on the organization's leadership philosophy. The context of the learning environment, including the support of key stakeholders, can influence NPD teaching and communication strategies, access to resources, and ability to effect change such as implementation of online learning.

Traditionally, NPD educators relied heavily on classroom teaching for employee orientation and other content-dense courses. Classes can vary in length from an hour to an all-day workshop or even to a multiple-session program. Shorter unit-based in-services can be useful for updating staff on new equipment, policies, or practices. Face-to-face teaching methods have been popular in staff development education for decades but have lost favor and practicality as the clinical environment becomes busier and more complicated than ever before (Haggard, 2011). In-service attendance has declined significantly as staffing models become leaner, and carving out even 15 to 30 minutes away from patient care can be difficult. Attendees are often interrupted with texts, alarms, and calls, leading to a chaotic learning environment. Other common education delivery methods in NPD include posters, videos, case studies, demonstration/redemonstration, self-learning packets, mobile learning carts, walking rounds, drop-in or open training sessions, proctored computer or skills labs, simulation, one-on-one precepting, pre- and posttests, surveys, demonstrations, journal clubs, and grand round presentations. Online and blended learning formats gained acceptance as viable strategies in recent years and are now a mainstay in many settings, providing much needed creative alternatives to traditional instructional approaches. Each of these methods has pros and cons for instructors and learners. As always, the choice of teaching strategy depends on subject matter, objectives, audience, time, resources, educator skill, and learners' preferred styles (Buchwach & Hill, 2017).

LEARNING THEORY CONSIDERATIONS

NPD practice is built on the principles of adult learning (Harper & Maloney, 2016). Coupled with constructivist learning theory, adult learning principles also anchor the approach to online teaching for nurses and other clinical staff. Central concepts of constructivist theory include interaction and collaborations along with reflection and experiential learning. Nurses build on the knowledge and experience they already have as they create or construct new meaning. NPD educators need to consider how nurses and others learn and be sure online materials and exercises are accessible, engaging, relevant, and practical. Content must be built using credible evidence and delivered in the right "dose," using the right terminology, and at the right level to connect with learners. Learners must actively engage in the education process to build meaning that they can use right away in real-world situations. In terms of course design and delivery, nurses expect clear directions, flexibility, self-pacing, intuitive navigation, logical progression, and easy access to resources as needed. And yes, learners appreciate when learning is also entertaining! When practical content is presented along with the chance to discover new information and get feedback on learning activities, learning and learner satisfaction are enhanced.

MANAGING LEARNING IN NPD

Employed in the right situations, online learning strategies allow NPD practitioners to reach learners quickly and conveniently. NPD pioneer Belinda Puetz (1991) envisioned this impact decades ago, claiming that using technology in staff development would be essential for productivity, efficiency, and cost-effectiveness. NPD educators tackle topics ranging from unit-specific equipment changes to yearly competency assessment for clinical staff to Joint Commission updates for all hospital employees. Each of these is unique and requires NPD educators to assess and validate needs, plan content and strategies, provide education, and evaluate the effectiveness of the program and the process itself. This is not a simple task. It takes time and money—resources that are already strained in a dynamic learning environment.

LMSs help educators to manage the "three Rs" of system-wide education efforts—registration, routing, and reporting (Dumpe, Kanyok, & Hill, 2007). Registration refers to assigning the right people to the right course or learning module and is usually done via job title or job code. Educators and stakeholders decide who the right people are at the outset of a project. Decisions are based on need, relevance, and appropriateness of the material. All staff, for example, may need customer service training, whereas only nurses, providers, and pharmacists may need modules on managing blood transfusion reactions. Routing refers to access and decisions about how, when, and where courses will be open and available to learners. Reporting is the important process of tracking attendance, performance, and completion rates of learners from specific roles or areas. Registration and tracking of online learning has become more sophisticated and reliable with improved system connectivity and secure cloud storage of information. These data are used for course management, employee performance appraisals, and regulatory recordkeeping. One hospital built and implemented an electronic system to track and monitor orientation and ongoing competency of their elite pediatric nurse transport team, saving them time and helping to ensure constant preparedness (Hickerson et al., 2018). In a technology survey of the Association for Nursing Professional Development (ANPD) members, 78% of respondents used a commercial or homegrown LMS to assign, deliver, store, track, and evaluate learning (Harper, Durkin, Orthoefer, Powers, & Tassinari, 2014). Accessibility, consistency, and tracking ability were listed as benefits of using an LMS, while complexity, cumbersome processes, and time to learn were noted as challenges.

INCORPORATING ONLINE STRATEGIES IN PROFESSIONAL SETTINGS

Competency Management

Maintaining nurse competency is a monumental undertaking, particularly as technology influences practice at full speed. Many hours of educator and staff time are involved, increasing the potential use of overtime funds and driving up costs. Competency validation in the past has been an extremely labor- and paper-intensive endeavor, often taking place in the form of multiple daylong "fairs" involving learning stations and manual signing of individual checklists. Online technology to demonstrate competency for nurses in the acute care environment has been used successfully. One five-site system with a goal of standardizing its annual chemotherapy competencies across all sites created a blended education program using online open-book test and learning resources and hands-on validation (Carreon, Sugarman, Beener, & Agan, 2015). Their efforts resulted in standardization of the policy, process, and equipment as well as lower costs and higher nurse confidence.

Preceptor Preparation

Another example demonstrating the usefulness of online education in NPD involves nurse preceptor preparation. Preceptors, experienced nurses who guide new nurses through orientation, need education and support in this role, which is performed in addition to their patient care responsibilities. Finding adequate and convenient time to educate preceptors without disrupting patient care is a challenge for NPD educators. Phillips (2006) suggested over a decade ago that online preceptor education programs could help preceptors quickly learn the role. There are many examples of online preceptor education since then. One fully online multiagency program comprised 10 online modules with discussion groups and online exercises. It was well received, and participants felt overall that learning online was a good option for preceptor preparation (Wink & Ruland, 2016). Online preceptor training programs have been successful in preparing certified registered nurse anesthetist (CRNA) and nurse practitioner preceptors as well (Easton, O'Donnell, Morrison, & Lutz, 2017; Wilkinson, Turner, Ellis, Knestrick, & Bondmass, 2015). Convenience and access are the main attractions of online learning for preceptors, and some suggest that the outcomes of an effective preceptor program, namely job satisfaction, retention, and recognition, can be met using online learning strategies.

Orientation

The activity that consumes perhaps the most NPD educator time is new employee orientation. Depending on the size of the organization, orientation takes place once or twice a month and can range from 1 day to 2 full weeks of face-to-face classroom or blended teaching strategies. Incorporating online learning strategies shortens the length of hospital orientation time significantly. Many organizations employ a blended approach, providing new employees with online information about the hospital mission and vision, benefits, review materials and tests, corporate compliance training, human resources policy links, and other general information for their review prior to starting a new job. NPD educators can also provide resources to help newly hired nurses prepare for a standard prehire medication calculation test. In such one instance, test scores improved dramatically (Payne, 2012). Classroom lecture time is decreased, and time can be used instead to meet team members and supervisors, clarify questions, practice skills, and review key points. Virtual or e-classrooms allow educators to deliver a consistent quality program built on information specific to the organization. Use of an online classroom modality where learners collaborate online both synchronously and asynchronously is driven by the need for more and more classroom time to cover material deemed mandatory or critical for new employees. Online learning provides a way for educators to cover more material without adding additional time or costs. Depending on hospital policy, some prework can be done before employees report for orientation or outside the hospital, decreasing the need for class time. Precious classroom interaction is used to clarify information and address learners' questions. Using online resources for orientation provides anytime access and allows for quick updating and revision of materials as changes occur. Printing costs are decreased, and training materials are easier to manage. For example, NPD can provide new employees with downloadable handouts and relevant intranet or Internet links instead of a full hardcover binder of printed material. Electronic checklists are not lost, are shareable among preceptors, and can easily be stored and filed. Although the online approach to orientation takes significant instructor time to design, build, test, upload, and manage, it eventually saved a great deal of time for both users and educators.

Continuing Education

Opportunities to incorporate online learning in NPD abound beyond new employee orientation. CE is a key component of nursing practice and, as such, often falls under the auspices of NPD. NPD educators are expected to create and provide creative, stimulating, up-to-date, cost-effective CE programs. Examples of CE include specialty courses such as breastfeeding certification preparation or advanced critical care courses, both of which are content rich and well suited for reconceptualization to online formats. These durable courses are reviewed and offered annually or as the need arises. Other applications include national online journal clubs using web-conferencing technology and live or recorded webinars for monthly topics with continuing nursing education (CNE) contact hours awarded to participants. NPD educators need to advocate for transformation of courses to online formats to strengthen the acceptance of technology-based learning for future endeavors. ANPD launched a successful national leadership academy (2017) and used web-based technology to house syllabi and other resources and to communicate with mentors and mentees in real time.

Mandatory Training

There are other examples of how online learning influences NPD practice. Annual mandatory training in fire safety, infection control, and corporate compliance can be translated with relative ease to an online format with the factual and standard nature of the content. All employees, volunteers, and students must complete the modules annually to comply with regulatory standards. Placing "mandatories" online and using an LMS for assigning, tracking, and reporting employee compliance results in real time is more efficient than offering multiple in-person classes and ensures that all staff get consistent information. Consideration must be made for follow-up and resource identification in the event of questions. Support for nonreaders or non–English-speaking learners must also be addressed, such as planning for a small number of face-to-face classes for each shift or making audio-assisted or transcript captioned versions of the learning module available. Accommodations must also be made for participants with disabilities. Specifics related to accommodating online learners are discussed in Chapter 11, Course Management Methods.

Some skill-based training has been converted to blended offerings as well. For example, the American Heart Association offers cardiopulmonary resuscitation (CPR) and advanced cardiac life support (ACLS) training for various user levels (bystander, professional) using a blended learning approach via their e-learning platform (American Heart Association, 2018). Learners register for and complete didactic content online and are then required to pass an instructor-led skills session using a voice-assisted manikin (VAM) to complete the course and receive a completion card. Instructor time is drastically reduced from approximately 4 hours per class to 1 hour per skills validation session, and learners can access and interact with the material at their convenience. Depending on setting and hospital policy, CPR and ACLS certifications are annual or biannual events, necessitating massive amounts of time, space, materials, and instruction when using a traditional face-to-face format. Serwetnyk et al. (2015) found that using online versus traditional methods for basic life support renewal classes saved time and money while maintaining staff confidence, satisfaction, and, most importantly, learning outcomes.

Collaboration

Online formats are also useful for sharing best practices, policies and procedures, blogs, and other collaborative documents. They are extremely helpful when working with students. Students must be welcomed and oriented to the clinical site and its electronic documentation system before starting their learning experience. They also have practical needs such as badging and security information. Large teaching hospital systems can feasibly host over a thousand students per year, and the use of online resources can dramatically reduce orientation time and instructor demand, not to mention mailing costs, redundancy, and misplaced documentation. The LMS can provide a way for students from several different programs to complete needed education such as Health Insurance Portability and Accountability Act (HIPAA) or cultural competency before arriving for their clinical experience, allowing them to focus on patient care once they arrive.

Online learning has usefulness outside the hospital setting as well. Nursing staff working in clinic or community settings also require education. It is impractical to arrange in-services and track attendance for staff who work across large geographic areas, require travel time, and manage unpredictable patient caseloads. Online formats can allow nurses and other clinicians to access and participate in webinars and other learning events without leaving their worksite. This is particularly useful in rural areas or settings without access to universities, experts, and other cutting-edge resources. In New York, nurse educators at a school of nursing worked with NPD educators and cancer center staff to develop a sophisticated online training program for patient navigators. Patient navigators are individuals who help guide patients and families through the complexities of care. Digital badges were awarded along the way as learners worked through content (Rohan, Fullerton, Escallier, & Pati, 2017).

With all its potential uses, online learning is not an automatic answer or silver bullet for all classes. NPD educators must still be mindful to appropriately align content and teaching strategies. As some online learning is static and one way, sensitive issues such as intimate partner violence or end-of-life care may not be best suited for an all-online format, particularly if presented in self-learning modules or if learners and instructor are present asynchronously. If sensitive topics are going to be offered online, they should be presented with an opportunity for discussion.

DECISION POINTS FOR USE OF ONLINE LEARNING STRATEGIES IN NPD

Stakeholders must make thoughtful and timely decisions about which teaching strategies will best meet learners' needs. After determining objectives and learning outcomes, cost issues and efficiency are urgent concerns. Time frames are often tight and must coincide with new regulations or changes in practice and equipment. Employees can be overwhelmed with the amount and frequency of information they are expected to absorb. In hospital environments, it is common for several education efforts to be underway simultaneously, creating multiple competing priorities. This can then lead to confusion, frustration, or even learner apathy. Getting the right information to the right employees at the right time and in the right way is critical, particularly in matters of patient safety or regulatory changes.

In recent years, electronic documentation "go lives" or enhancements have been extremely complex for trainers and stressful for staff. Of note, the Association of American Medical Colleges claims that electronic health records (EHRs) are a leading contributor to widespread physician burnout (Breining, 2018). Some organizations have even called upon the Institute for Healthcare Improvement (IHI) to add a fourth, or quadruple, aim of care team well-being to the Triple Aims of patient experience, population health, and reducing costs (Lippincott Solutions, 2017). This is mentioned as learner stress and patient safety are constants in the context of learning in a professional setting, regardless of the chosen format.

Supervisors and managers struggle with schedules and unit budgets, which can become burdened when employees attend class during or in addition to their regular work hours. Make-up sessions for "no show" employees put pressure on educators and further impact the bottom line. For these reasons, online learning options are attractive for the flexibility and scope they offer.

Other factors also contribute to the decision to go online. Depending on the generality of the content and objectives, purchase of an "out of the box" education product may be a sound option. For hospital- or unit-specific material, a pediatric unit's security and visitation policy, for example, it may be more appropriate to develop online materials in-house. Purchase of ready-made materials may save time but can be cost-prohibitive depending on licensure policies for multiple users. Relevance or shelf life of learning products should also be considered as policies and practice change rapidly. In-house materials may save money but can take weeks or months to develop, pilot, and deliver to the learners who need the information. One alternative is to purchase ready-made modules with options for customization, which allows educators to add or edit content to reflect hospital policies and processes.

Other considerations for using online modalities include educator proficiency and comfort with technology, space and instructor availability, stakeholder support and buy-in, learner acceptance of online learning, and availability of information technology infrastructure and support. Harper and Maloney (2016) found that NPD practitioners were not using technology to its full potential and charged them to develop their individual competence in educational technologies, including online learning. In the end, whether online, blended, or more traditional methods are chosen, it is most important that solid education design and delivery align to help learners meet their goals.

FACILITATORS AND BARRIERS TO USE OF ONLINE LEARNING IN NPD

As stated throughout this chapter, there are recognized facilitators and barriers to the use of online learning in clinical settings. Factors that support the use of online learning include flexibility and convenience of scheduling and the ability to reach lots of learners in a short time. Cost savings are realized through decreased class time, which translates to fewer "nonproductive" salary dollars and less need for instructor, space, and printed resources. Learners can easily access online learning resources at their convenience, and LMSs help educators manage registration, routing, and reporting. From a design perspective, materials can be efficiently updated or revised to reflect current standards and practices as changes occur. NPD educators can design modules to appeal to various learning levels and styles and to adhere to the adult learning principles of relevance, independent learning, and applicability to real life. Most millennial, Gen Y, and Gen Z learners are digital natives and are accustomed to all things electronic, so online learning does not constitute a barrier in terms of learning in the workplace.

Along with these advantages, there are certain barriers to successful use of online learning in NPD. From a learner standpoint, barriers may include inadequate computing skills, particularly when digital immigrants are expected to learn new content and new technology at the same time, or limited access to computers or courseware. Some staff may resist a change in how education is delivered, preferring a more traditional classroom or face-to-face approach. From an organizational standpoint, a lack of devices, connectivity, software, or information technology support for designing and building usable programs may create administrative bottlenecks and negative perceptions of online learning. From an environmental standpoint, noisy stressful work areas, which are commonplace in hospitals, can hamper the online learning experience.

NPD educators themselves, if not skilled in or supportive of online learning, may inadvertently be barriers to learning. Poorly designed, outdated, haphazard online learning materials will quickly lead to learner disengagement and poor learning outcomes. Educators unfamiliar with online teaching strategies should seek out available resources such as SMEs, library personnel, faculty partners, and instructional design experts to ensure that materials are appropriate and well conceptualized for online learning. Modules or courses should be piloted and revised as needed before being assigned to live users. There are also formal academic courses for NPD educators who desire to improve their online teaching skills. For example, the Institute for Educators at the University of Maryland School of Nursing offers a 3-credit online graduate level course in teaching in online environments and face-to-face workshops for educators in all settings (UMSON, 2018).

Perhaps a less obvious barrier is an inconsistency of NPD educators to clearly convey outcomes and return on investment (ROI) of online learning projects. Without compelling data to support new approaches to learning, NPD educators risk losing the opportunity to fully leverage online learning and its many benefits. In 2018, ANPD launched an online ROI calculator to help NPD educators project costs, break-even points, and estimated savings based on the results of educational efforts.

MEASUREMENT OF OUTCOMES

According to the ANA Scope and Standards of Practice for NPD (Harper & Maloney, 2016), educators "formulate a systematic and effective evaluation plan aimed at measuring processes and outcomes that are relevant to the program, learners, and stakeholders" (p. 41). Owing to time constraints and the challenge of following up with learners in a shifting environment, programs are not consistently evaluated beyond the level of a "happy sheet" or postclass learner evaluation. Historically, NPD educators rigorously track the number of sessions, attendees, and CE contact hours related to a course. They collect test scores and learner satisfaction surveys to determine the outcome of classes or courses. But to truly make a case for the benefits of an education effort, and specifically the ROI for online learning strategies, NPD educators are encouraged to set outcome criteria at the outset of a program and fully engage in the evaluation process. By determining desired outcomes at the outset of a project (i.e., fewer patient falls, decreased catheter infection rates, improved compliance with medication reconciliation), NPD educators can partner with stakeholders to develop a comprehensive evaluation plan. Outcomes related to education can be evaluated via quality improvement and risk management data, chart audits, feedback from participants and stakeholders, and human resources or financial data. For example, to evaluate the value of a new online fall safety program, NPD educators might compare the cost of new learning technology and software license fees against the cost savings of instructor time, employee salaries, materials, and, ultimately, a decrease in patient length of stay due to a decrease in falls.

The Kirkpatrick four-level model of program evaluation has been called a "classic in the industry" of NPD (Warren, 2009) and is useful in program evaluation. Its four distinct levels of evaluation help to determine program effectiveness and value (Kirkpatrick & Kirkpatrick, 2006; Standish & Dickerson, 2017). The first level, called *reaction*, assesses whether learners are satisfied with the program from a delivery perspective. Questions may include the following: Were the instructions clear? Was the content interesting and easily accessible? Was the program length correct? Level two, *learning*, asks if learners achieved what they intended to from the program. Did they achieve stated objectives? Did they learn what they expected to learn? The first two levels can usually be assessed at the time of the training. In an online environment, learners might be asked to complete an evaluation survey before exiting the course or receiving a certificate. *Behavior* is the third level of evaluation in Kirkpatrick's model, and it assesses whether the new learning "sticks" over time. In other words, can nurses implement fall precautions and document appropriately 1 month after the training? Can they state fall safety protocols? Level four, *results* or *impact*, looks "down the line" to see if the change has had a positive impact on the system or organization. Educators could use risk management data to determine the number and rate of falls compared to the preprogram data. Because levels three and four take time and require detailed follow-up, they may not be done as consistently as levels one and two. This model is straightforward yet flexible and could easily be applied to the evaluation of online learning programs in NPD. Use of this or a similar evaluation model to collect evaluation data can add considerable credibility to NPD practice and help solidify the ROI case for incorporation of online learning strategies. Evaluation data also enhance credibility and aid in dissemination of best practices.

RESEARCH OPPORTUNITIES

There has been remarkable growth in the use of online learning in NPD. Looking back, a National Nursing Staff Development Organization's (NNSDO) position statement from 2006 did not mention the use of online learning as an NPD teaching strategy. Rather, its focus was on online learning as an academic option, but NPD supported distance learning as a viable vehicle for learning. By 2009, the Core Curriculum for Staff Development (Bruce, 2009) included a chapter on using technology, and by 2010, the NNSDO Public Policy Agenda (NNSDO, 2010) committed to supporting education-based research and the use of new pedagogies and technology to connect to nursing practice. In the most recent Core Curriculum for NPD, the technology chapter includes subtopics on using technology in NPD practice and in online environments (Brady-Schluttner, 2017). Teaching technology and online learning are now hardwired into NPD practice and competencies.

Examples of online learning and technology-related teaching strategies are plentiful in the practice and CE literature as outlined in this chapter. Hospitals use online learning platforms for all phases of the teaching process, and the use is anticipated to increase as interprofessional and team learning activities gain popularity and as Baby Boomers retire from the workplace. The potential applications for online learning are boundless. Sherman, Comer, Putnam, and Freeman (2012) found no significant difference in nurses' learning outcomes or learner satisfaction scores between blended learning and lecture approaches to pharmacology education. Pilcher and Bedford (2011) found that nurses of all ages indicated a willingness to learn using various technological tools. Ease of use, familiarity, convenience, and perceived benefit were the key determinants of their willingness to do so. NPD educators should be sure to use evidence when advocating for online learning approaches.

Research evidence on the direct translation of online knowledge to nursing practice is sparse but is gaining attention and momentum, particularly from an ROI perspective. NPD educators and executive stakeholders alike should focus on the "down the line" impact of all educational activities, including online learning. They must question the outcomes on patient care and other measurable clinical outcomes. Until recently, much evidence about the effectiveness of online learning involved students. Little research existed regarding the impact of an online learning environment on practicing nurses. What evidence there was involved small sample sizes and was not generalizable.

Recently, ANPD identified 10 focus areas for the specialty's spirit of inquiry, which encompasses research, evidence-based practice, and quality improvement studies and projects (Harper, Warren, Bradley, Bindon, & Maloney, 2018). The project team solicited input from three groups including NPD conference attendees, NPD leaders, and the society journal's editorial board members. Use of teaching technology and online learning figured prominently in the feedback from all groups. The final 10 priorities align with the NPD Practice Model (Harper & Maloney, 2016) and include strategies that significantly increase engagement of learners and types of technology that enhance learning (throughput) and development of learning outcomes metrics (outputs). Work in these areas of inquiry will further describe and inform NPD practitioners about the creative use and benefits of online learning in professional practice.

FUTURE

The role of learning technology and potential use of online education by NPD educators in clinical settings is limitless. Looking ahead, Bindon (2016, p. 351) predicted that "technology will affect every aspect of NPD practice" and that education will be more and more "individualized, mobile, nimble, flexible, and accessible on demand."

We can anticipate NPD educators debriefing interprofessional practice scenarios in virtual clinical areas, mobile clinical resources, increased use of smart technology, enhanced online partnerships and mentoring with schools of nursing and other professions, and greater online interaction between patients and the healthcare team. Its actual use will evolve at varying paces in different settings, limited by educator experience with online teaching strategies, organizational decisions regarding whether enhancements to online learning resources is a worthwhile venture, learner acceptance and competence, user sophistication, and technical support to make the online learning experience effective and satisfying.

The responsibility for demonstrating that online learning strategies can produce a strong ROI in terms of cost and time savings and improved patient and organizational outcomes lies with NDP educators. Educators must continue to respect and uphold high educational standards in the design and delivery of online content (Gormley, 2013). This will be done via a thoughtful, outcomes-based approach to learning needs assessment, course design, learning engagement, and program evaluation.

SUMMARY

This chapter focuses on the utility and effectiveness of online and technology-supported learning in clinical settings. The chapter includes an overview of the role of clinical nurse educators, known as NPD practitioners, and their pivotal role in supporting professional, ancillary staff, and student learning needs in a clinical setting. The learning environment itself poses unique challenges in a busy healthcare setting, and these are described as well. Several applications of online learning, including clinical orientation, preceptor preparation, competency management, and delivery of mandatory training and regulatory updates, are presented. There are benefits and challenges when implementing online education for learners, instructors, and organizational stakeholders alike. Integral to the success of online and technology-supported learning in the clinical setting is a solid foundation in adult learning principles, sound educational design, and thoughtful decision-making by all involved. Consistent evaluation of ROI is a key factor in the ongoing success and adoption of online learning in the future of NPD.

REFERENCES

American Heart Association. (2018, October). *Emergency cardiovascular care.* Retrieved from https://cpr.heart.org/AHAECC/CPRAndECC/FindACourse/CourseFormats/UCM_473163_Course-Formats.jsp

American Nurses Association. (2014). *Position statement on professional role competence.* Washington, DC: American Nurses Association. Retrieved from https://www.nursingworld.org/practice-policy/nursing-excellence/official-position-statements/id/professional-role-competence

American Nurses Credentialing Center. (2018). *Nursing professional development certification test content outline.* Retrieved from https://www.nursingworld.org/~4acbba/globalassets/certification/certification-specialty-pages/resources/test-content-outlines/nursingprofessionaldevelopment-tco.pdf

Bindon, S. L. (2016). Future nursing professional development services and focus. In C. M. Smith & M. G. Harper (Ed.), *Leadership in nursing professional development: An organizational and system focus* (pp. 332–355). Chicago, IL: Association for Nursing Professional Development.

Bindon, S. L. (2017). Professional development strategies to enhance nurses' knowledge and maintain safe practice. *AORN Journal, 106*(2), 99–110. doi:10.1016/j.aorn.2017.06.002

Brady-Schluttner, K. (2017). Technology in nursing professional development. In P. S. Dickerson (Ed.), *Core curriculum for nursing professional development* (5th ed., pp. 160–169). Chicago, IL: Association for Nursing Professional Development.

Breining, G. (2018). Reducing stress associated with electronic health record. *AAMC News.* Retrieved from https://news.aamc.org/patient-care/article/reducing-stress-electronic-health-records

Bruce, S. L. (Ed.). (2009). *Core curriculum for staff development* (3rd ed.). Pensacola, FL: National Nursing Staff Development Organization.

Buchwach, D., & Hill, L. (2017). Teaching methodologies and learner engagement. In P. S. Dickerson (Ed.), *Core curriculum for nursing professional development* (5th ed., pp. 134–158). Chicago, IL: Association for Nursing Professional Development.

Carreon, N., Sugarman, C., Beener, E., & Agan, D. (2015). Creating and standardizing annual chemotherapy competencies throughout a healthcare system. *Journal for Nurses in Professional Development, 31*(1), 35–39. doi:10.1097/NND.0000000000000131

Chicca, J., & Shellenbarger, T. (2018). Connecting with generation Z: Approaches in nursing education. *Teaching and Learning in Nursing, 13*(3), 180–184. doi:10.1016/j.teln.2018.03.008

Dumpe, M. L., Kanyok, N., & Hill, K. (2007). Use of an automated learning management system to validate nursing competencies. *Journal for Nurses in Staff Development, 23*(4), 183–185. doi:10.1097/01.NND.0000281418.50472.2e

Easton, A., O'Donnell, J., Morrison, S., & Lutz, C. (2017). Development of an online, evidence-based CRNA preceptor training tutorial (CPiTT): A quality improvement project. *AANA Journal, 85*(5), 331–339. Retrieved from https://www.aana.com/docs/default-source/aana-journal-web-documents-1/development-online-1017-pp331-339pdf.pdf?sfvrsn=652d45b1_6

Gormley, D. K. (2013). Considerations when developing online continuing education programs in nursing. *Journal for Nurses in Professional Development, 29*(3), 149–151. doi:10.1097/NND.0b013e318291c47d

Haggard, A. (2011). Unit inservice classes—Are they obsolete? *Journal for Nurses in Staff Development, 27*(6), 301–303. doi:10.1097/NND.0b013e31823864e5

Harper, M. G., Durkin, G., Orthoefer, D. K., Powers, R., & Tassinari, R. M. (2014). ANPD technology survey: The state of NPD practice. *Journal for Nurses in Professional Development, 30*(5), 242–247. doi:10.1097/NND.0000000000000106

Harper, M. G., & Maloney, P. (Eds.). (2016). *Nursing professional development: Scope and standards of practice* (3rd ed.). Chicago, IL: Association for Nursing Professional Development.

Harper, M. G., Warren, J. I., Bradley, D., Bindon, S. L., & Maloney, P. (2018). Nursing professional development's spirit of inquiry focus areas. *Journal for Nurses in Professional Development.* Advance online publication. doi:10.1097/NND.0000 000000000515

Hickerson, K., Agosto, P., Cieplinski, J. A., Hutchins, L., Squires, L., & Tsarouhas, N. (2018). A transparent tracking system for competency-based orientation: One children's hospital transport unit experience. *Journal for Nurses in Professional Development, 34*(3), 173–177. doi:10.1097/NND.0000000000000422

Kirkpatrick, D. L., & Kirkpatrick, J. D. (2006). *Evaluating training programs: The four levels* (3rd ed.). San Francisco, CA: Berrett-Koehler.

Lippincott Solutions. (2017). *Moving from triple to quadruple aim* [Blog post]. Retrieved from http://lippincottsolutions.lww.com/blog.entry.html/2017/09/05/moving _from_triplet-uouA.html

National Nursing Staff Development Organization. (2010). *Nursing professional development: Scope and standards of practice.* Silver Spring, MD: American Nurses Association.

Payne, L. (2012). Electronic classroom: Supporting nursing education. *Journal for Nurses in Staff Development, 6,* 292–293. doi:10.1097/NND.0b013e318274b102

Phillips, J. M. (2006). Preparing preceptors through online education. *Journal for Nurses in Staff Development, 22*(3), 150–156. doi:10.1097/00124645-200605000-00010

Pilcher, J. W., & Bedford, L. (2011). Willingness and preferences of nurses related to learning with technology. *Journal for Nurses in Staff Development, 27*(3), E10–E16. doi:10.1097/NND.0b013e318217b447

Puetz, B. (1991). Getting ourselves computerized [Editorial]. *Journal for Nurses in Professional Development, 7*(2), 59–60. Retrieved from https://journals.lww.com/jnsdonline/Citation/1991/03000/Getting_Ourselves_Computerized.1.aspx

Rheingans, J. (2016). The nursing professional development practice model. *Journal for Nurses in Professional Development, 32*(5), 278–281. doi:10.1097/NND.0000000000000283

Rohan, A. J., Fullerton, J. Escallier, L. A., & Pati, S. (2017). Creating a novel online digital badge-awarding program in patient navigation to address healthcare access. *Journal for Nurses in Professional Development, 33*(3), 106–112. doi:10.1097/NND.0000000000000357

Serwetnyk, T. M., Filmore, K., VonBacho, S., Cole, R., Miterko, C., Smith, C., & Smith, C. M. (2015). Comparison on online and traditional basic life support renewal training methods for registered professional nurses. *Journal for Nurses in Professional Development, 31*(6), E1–E10. doi:10.1097/NND.0000000000000201

Shanley, C. (2004). Extending the role of nurses in staff development by combining an organizational change perspective with an individual learner perspective. *Journal for Nurses in Staff Development, 20*(2), 83–89.

Sherman, H., Comer, L., Putnam, L., & Freeman, H. (2012). Blended versus lecture learning: Outcomes for staff development. *Journal for Nurses in Professional Development, 28*(4), 186–190. doi:10.1097/NND.0b013e31825dfb71

Standish, C., & Dickerson, P. (2017). Establishing measurable outcomes for educational activities and departments. In P. S. Dickerson (Ed.), *Core curriculum for nursing professional development* (5th ed., pp. 114–125). Chicago, IL: Association for Nursing Professional Development.

University of Maryland School of Nursing. (2018, October). *Teaching in nursing and health professions.* Retrieved from http://www.nursing.umaryland.edu/academics/certificates/teaching

Valentine, C. M. (2018). Tackling the quadruple aim: Helping cardiovascular professionals find work-life balance. *Journal of the American College of Cardiology, 71*(15), 1707–1709. doi:10.1016/j.jacc.2018.03.014

Warren, J. I. (2009). Program evaluation/return on investment. In S. L. Bruce (Ed.), *Core curriculum for staff development* (3rd ed., pp. 297–320). Pensacola, FL: National Nursing Staff Development Organization.

Wilkinson, M., Turner, B., Ellis, K., Knestrick, J., & Bondmass, M. (2015). Online clinical education training for preceptors: A pilot QI project. *The Journal for Nurse Practitioners, 11*(7), 43–50. doi:10.1016/j.nurpra.2015.04.017

Wink, D., & Ruland, J. (2016). Multiagency online preceptor education: Design, implementation, and outcomes. *Nurse Educator, 41*(5), 270–273. doi:10.1097/NNE.0000000000000261

Wolters Kluwer Health. (2014). *Wolters Kluwer Health survey finds nurses and healthcare institutions accepting professional use of online reference & mobile technology.* Retrieved from https://wolterskluwer.com/company/newsroom/news/health/2014/09/wolters-kluwer-health-survey-finds-nurses-and-healthcare-institutions-accepting-professional-use-of-online-reference--mobile-technology.html

Wright, D. (2005). *The ultimate guide to competency assessment in health care* (3rd ed.). Minneapolis, MN: Creative Health Care Management.

9

Theoretical Applications of Continuing Education

William A. Sadera and Kathleen A. Gould

INTRODUCTION

The availability of technology-supported continuing education (CE) for medical professionals emerged in the early 1990s. Since that time, physicians, nurses, and other healthcare professionals have continued to seek available technology-supported CE because of the convenience, accessibility, and flexibility that it affords the users. Online and distance learning technologies are not new, but the increased capabilities and potential to reach a larger audience have transformed how we deliver education and training. More importantly, it has expanded our capacity to respond to the need to keep health professionals' knowledge and experiences current. With a long history of serving isolated and remote learners, distance learning is now commonplace and accepted as an effective, mainstream delivery method of education and training that provides flexible learning opportunities in response to the needs of learners. Because of the wide acceptance of online distance learning, it is important to consider appropriate pedagogical methods for delivering effective distance-based CE.

Historically, the results of research on effective distance learning pedagogy have been ignored and have not been applied to CE courses. Although the findings of empirical studies are essential to the quality of the distance learning experience, administrators and faculty have only recently started to apply the results. This chapter provides an overview of distance-based CE as well as current theoretical approaches to online learning in CE. The purpose of this chapter is to review the current best practices and discuss the application of sound pedagogy, effective design, and the theoretical approaches that inform the design.

DISTANCE-BASED CE

With the rapid expansion of CE offerings online, it is becoming imperative that sound pedagogical design and the integration of emerging technologies be appropriately applied to the learning environment. With the realization that lifelong learning is more than attending conferences, the potential for greatly expanding effective continuing medical education (CME) through online learning technologies has never been more encouraging. Because the primary audience for CE comprises busy, working adult learners, institutions should ideally show consideration for these learners so that they have a choice in the organization and delivery of the learning program. Specifically, the aim of most CE is to help improve practices and behaviors to provide the best quality care to patients and to maintain currency in practice. Nurses and physicians specifically require CE for acquiring new knowledge, skills, and attitudes that must be learned to keep pace with changes in practice. Traditional continuing professional education is taught through passive activities, such as lectures, face-to-face classes, and seminars. This kind of professional education usually requires the participants to be in the same place at the same time, which often does not coincide with the time demands of busy, working professionals.

Given the factors addressed through the guidance of learning theory, combined with the convenience and flexibility afforded through online education, offerings in this format will only continue to increase. Along with the increasing demand and growing consumer experience with distance learning modalities, expectations for quality instruction, successful educational outcomes, and satisfying learning experiences will also increase. Therefore, it is imperative to examine and compare the most effective methods of delivering CME.

Mazzoleni, Maugeri, Rognoni, Cantoni, and Imbriani (2012) started an online educational program aimed at evaluating the impact of healthcare staff attendance as well as objective and subjective effectiveness. In a 15-month time frame, five e-learning courses were provided to 2,261 potential users at 14 hospitals, in parallel with traditional education. One thousand ninety-nine users from all 14 hospitals attended the courses (58% of nurses, 50% of therapists, 44% of technicians, 25% of physicians) for a total of 27,459 CME credits. Effectiveness, in terms of knowledge gain, was satisfactory, as was subjective evaluation of the e-learning courses (more than 95% were satisfied users). E-learning is not always appropriate for all educational needs and is not a panacea, but the reported results point out that it may be an effective and economically convenient solution to support massive educational interventions, reaching results otherwise not attainable with traditional education (Mazzoleni et al., 2012).

In a review of 30 CE courses, quality of content was the characteristic most important to participants, and too little interaction was the largest source of dissatisfaction (Casebeer et al., 2004). The online environment provides numerous tools to promote communication and interaction that can allow learners to examine their own assumptions and develop new perspectives (Cahill, 2014). More current research into networking and interactivity among practitioners is providing new information that has the potential to enhance the effectiveness of practice improvement. Insights from learning theories can provide a framework for understanding emergent learning that results from interactions among individuals in trusted relationships such as online communities of practice. Failure to take advantage of practitioner interactivity may explain, in part, why some practice improvement study results show low rates of effectiveness. Examples of improvement models that explicitly use relationship building and facilitation techniques to enhance practitioner interactivity have demonstrated effectiveness (Jakubec, Parboosingh, & Colvin, 2014; Parboosingh, Reed, Caldwell, & Bernstein, 2011). Curricula to teach relationship building in communities of practice and facilitation skills to enhance learning in small group education sessions continue to be explored.

Other indications that interactivity and engagement may be key factors to successfully design CME have been described by Reed, Schifferdecker, and Turco (2012). These authors found that students who wrote personal learning plans as a part of their CME experience were "very close" or "extremely close" to accomplishing learning goals following the training. Additionally, Saba (2016) has suggested that social, cognitive, and teaching presence are important to online learning satisfaction. Teachers have an important role in providing guidance in an online community while learners have shifting roles and at times become teachers (Saba, 2016). These findings suggest that distance-based CE can be effective, but it is the design of these courses that needs to be scrutinized to ensure a successful learning experience. Reed et al. (2012) suggested that the integration of strategies to implement research-based pedagogy is necessary to ensure that practices change. The CE developers are responsible for responding to the needs of professionals to design, deliver, and evaluate new approaches to course design to determine the effectiveness of meeting the required outcomes.

Recent reviews of online CME instruction by Vannieuwenborg, Goossens, De Lepeleire, and Schoenmakers (2016) revealed that the most online CME delivery is still text based, followed by text and graphics, slide presentation or slides and audio, text and audio, or texts, articles, and questionnaires. Over past years, there continues to be an unsophisticated approach to CE design despite research findings; however, this approach is slowly beginning to change. For example, Pullen (2013) surveyed students in 42 CME courses and found that course formats that provided immediate feedback, allowed the learner to apply new knowledge to clinical- or question-type responses, and provided opportunities for active learning and autonomy or self-pacing were consistent with learner satisfaction. In addition, learning formats that replace static slide presentations with case studies or actor videos designed to mimic scenarios that would be encountered in a doctor's office have been successfully implemented to deliver CME (see med.stanford.edu/cme.html). Developing learning platforms that utilize digital technology to incorporate these interactive characteristics are vital to improving online CME.

CE AND QUALITY EDUCATION

As distance-based CE has grown steadily over the past several years, the quality has received limited attention in the medical literature, and few have attempted to establish or describe quality standards. Standards can be used to synthesize practical knowledge, best practices, and research findings. Sadly, they often vary in their perspectives on quality, fall short of being comprehensive, and convey many elements that apply to distance CE. The conclusions are that published standards in the distance education literature in general can provide valuable guidance to distance CE providers, and additional research questioning what works in CE and why is clearly needed. Standards, such as Quality Matters (see www.qualitymatters.org/qa-resources/rubric-standards/cpe-rubric), should be regarded as an instrument to achieve appropriate design decisions for online instruction and maintain high learning goals while remaining cognizant of what the program is trying to achieve.

A framework for implementing technology-enabled knowledge translation into the healthcare culture was described by Ho et al. (2004). They claimed that cultivation and acceptance in the domains of perceiving types of knowledge and ways in which clinicians acquire and apply knowledge in practice are required. Ho et al. (2004) argued that in order for knowledge transfer to take place, the following issues need to be met: understanding the conceptual and contextual frameworks of information and communication technologies as applied to healthcare systems; comprehending essential issues in implementation of information and communication technologies as well as strategies to take advantage of emerging opportunities; and, finally, establishing a common and widely acceptable evaluation framework. The successful transfer of knowledge from a technology-supported learning environment to practice, according to these authors, depends on a vision about the goals to be achieved, identification of cultural and political issues, and human and financial resources, as well as addressing legal, ethical, and technological limitations. This framework considered the complex elements of CE design coupled with technology and the ultimate purpose for delivery being that of change in practice.

New developments in technology allow today's CE providers to more effectively meet the criteria necessary for effective CE. These factors include convenience, relevance, individualization, self-assessment, independent learning, and a systematic approach to learning. A case study conducted at the International Virtual Medical Schools in the United Kingdom (Harden, 2005) demonstrated how rapid growth of distance learning can alter undergraduate education and can have the potential to alter the nature of CE. Key components include a bank of reusable learning objects, a virtual practice with virtual patients, a learning outcomes framework, and self-assessment instruments. Learning is facilitated by a curriculum map, guided learning resources, "ask the experts" opportunities, and collaboration or peer-to-peer learning. Harden also found that distance learning provided a bridge between the cutting edge of education and training and outdated procedures embedded in institutions and professional organizations. It is often these organizations that can be credited for keeping healthcare professionals up to date with current practice issues.

If healthcare professionals are not kept up to date with current practice, the design and subsequently the quality of CE course offerings are only going to deteriorate. Without the keen attention and deliberate actions for incorporating research findings into new course design, healthcare practitioners will ultimately not be able to achieve their goal of knowledge enhancement for the ultimate purpose of providing current, up-to-date patient care.

IMPROVING QUALITY OF CE

Better programs would not be possible without consideration of practitioner experiences that suggest that interacting with peers and mentors in the workplace provides the best environment for learning, which, in turn, enhances professional practice and professional judgment (Parboosingh et al., 2011). This assertion is supported by research findings that reaffirm two important principles in adult learning. First, we learn most naturally when faced with meaningful problem-solving experiences; second, learning results in action when constructed by the individual. Without sound pedagogical principles and theoretical considerations for interaction and learner experiences, quality distance CE will not be possible (Parboosingh et al., 2011). Although the trend is to put more and more CE online, it has only been recently that pedagogical considerations for design and delivery are starting to be noted (Fisher & Sadera, 2011).

Several key pedagogical considerations can be noted in the distance learning and CE literature based on the theoretical approaches discussed earlier. Although distance education programs enhance access to CE for the health professional, increased access is often coupled with decreased quality in course design. According to Carriere and Harvey (2001), good course quality must consider an understanding of the experiences of the providers. Because of this need for understanding, a web-based survey aimed at CE providers was constructed to elicit a description of the providers, users, and the activities offered. This study revealed that participants had considerable interest in distance education development. As distance CE features are now better known, this is a step toward the advancement and development of more and better distance programs as organizations share their experiences and models for programs. Online CE should incorporate interactive learning based on adult learning principles and facilitate the effective use of Web 2.0 tools. Furthermore, providers of CE should continue to investigate barriers that adults encounter pursuing online learning formats (Cahill, 2014). Dolcourt, Zuckerman, and Warner (2006) noted competing time demands, irrelevant topics, and inconveniences such as parking and inclement weather as major factors for poor attendance at CE offerings in traditional formats. Improved accessibility, affordability of distance education, and time efficiency compared to the traditional conference-type programs are often cited as the primary reasons for offering distance-based CE. CE providers are keenly aware of professionals' busy schedules and are trying to accommodate their needs by offering ease of access and time efficiency. As consumers of educational products, busy healthcare providers make choices among competing alternatives for their time. By recognizing key decision factors, CE developers can potentially increase attendance and satisfaction by structuring style, content, and logistics to better accommodate the learners' perspectives.

In recent years, CE developers were looking at interactive strategies to enhance learning using activities such as "blogging" or reflective journaling. A study by Bouldin, Homes, and Fortenberry (2006) found that although reflective journaling can be used as a learner-centered assessment tool to determine whether students are making sense of the content discussed in class, the students described this activity as "busy work." This demonstrates the need for interaction to be an integral part of the course design, not just an added activity. This notion was validated by a study in 2011 by Fisher and Sadera who found that if the mechanisms for interactivity are not integral (i.e., optional), then the learners are less likely to utilize them and therefore will not benefit.

Davis et al. (1999) reviewed randomized controlled trials on CE interventions and found personal interaction to be central to effective change in practice. Several studies reported that healthcare professionals seek confirmation and validation of current and new medical practices through their peers. For example, Jakubec et al. (2014) found that learners who actively participated in communities of practice perceived better acquisition of course objectives and enhanced benefits from course participation. Other studies have confirmed the importance of interaction in changing professional behavior. However, researchers have not established which elements of the interactive process enable learning. This is despite the preference shown among physician groups that many prefer lectures, although this may include interaction if it is built into the design of the class in a meaningful way to build knowledge.

Learning and practice cannot be separated when professionals work closely in specialty areas within the healthcare arena (Parboosingh et al., 2011). Interestingly, physicians report that such interactions with colleagues are an important source of learning, and educators and course designers have only recently considered using the power of communities to foster learning through practice (Parboosingh et al., 2011). Membership within a learning community, however, has its responsibilities, because expectations and pressures from peers and mentors in a community of practice influence standards for learning and practice. Jakubec et al. (2014) found that course participants who actively participated in communities of practice perceived greater success in meeting course objectives than those who were not as actively engaged. The significance of this finding tells us that continuing professional development providers should focus on meeting the learning needs of multidisciplinary communities of practice rather than individual learners. This research has implications for design considerations of CE courses.

Problem-solving strategies illustrate the contribution of theory to practice. The ability to frame and solve problems is central to the healthcare professional's level of competence. It is known that the ability to solve problems is tightly tied to one's knowledge in that area; therefore, problem-solving ability varies markedly from case to case and from context to context. These findings have led to new understandings and revised theories about promoting the learning of problem-solving. We now know that learners require a wide variety and number of opportunities along with exemplars in learning how to solve problems so that they have many different strategies and approaches in their arsenal. The iterative relationship between theory and practice provides a powerful tool for improvement in the field.

SUMMARY

The importance of technology to healthcare professional development is growing rapidly and is echoed throughout the literature. Access to distance CE must be immediate, relevant, credible, easy to use, cost efficient, and effective. A sense of high utility demands content that is focused and well indexed to meet the needs of healthcare professionals. The roles of the CE provider must continue to evolve to include strategies for helping healthcare professionals seek and construct the kind of knowledge they need to improve patient care.

Although developing, distance-based CE still lacks a theoretical underpinning, integration of best practices for teaching, and effective utilization of technology to enhance the quality of course offerings. If guided constructivism were used to design online learning environments, objectives would be learner centered and would help to guide the learning experience. Emphasis should be placed on the process of knowledge construction rather than on the outcomes of learning. Content should be presented to accommodate various learning styles and developmental levels, and an emphasis should be placed on active and experiential learning through questions, case studies, and projects that can help the student develop mental models and test reality. These approaches allow the student to apply basic information to real-world practice. Experimenting with your student population, instructional beliefs, and varied practices will help you find the best ways to design effective online instruction for your learner population. Current research should apply what is known from the field of educational research coupled with what is known about the health professional as a learner to deliver quality learning opportunities with better outcomes for practicing healthcare providers.

REFERENCES

Bouldin, A., Holmes, E., & Fortenberry, M. (2006). Blogging about course concepts: Using technology for reflective journaling in a communications course. *American Journal of Pharmaceutical Education, 70*(4), 84. doi:10.5688/aj700484

Cahill, J. (2014). How distance education has improved adult education. *The Educational Forum, 78*(3), 316–322. doi:10.1080/00131725.2014.912366

Carriere, M., & Harvey, D. (2001). Current state of distance continuing medical education in North America. *Journal of Continuing Education in the Health Professions, 21*, 150–157. doi:10.1002/chp.1340210305

Casebeer, L., Kristofco, R., Strasser, S., Reilly, M., Krishnamoorthy, P., Rabin, A., ... Myers, L. (2004). Standardizing evaluation of online continuing medical education: Physician knowledge, attitudes, and reflection on practice. *Journal of Continuing Education in the Health Professions, 24*, 68–75. doi:10.1002/chp.1340240203

Davis, D., O'Brien, M. A., Freemantle, N., Wolf, F. M., Mazmanian, P., & Taylor-Vaisey, A. (1999). Impact of formal continuing medical education: Do conferences, workshops, rounds, and other traditional continuing education activities change physician behavior or health care outcomes? *Journal of the American Medical Association, 282*(9), 867–874. doi:10.1001/jama.282.9

Dolcourt, J., Zuckerman, G., & Warner, K. (2006). Learners' decisions for attending pediatric grand rounds: A qualitative and quantitative study. *BMC Medical Education, 6*(26), 1–8. doi:10.1186/1472-6920-6-26

Fisher, C., & Sadera, W. (2011). Comparing student learning and satisfaction between learning environments in continuing medical education. *International Journal of Instructional Technology and Distance Learning, 8*(5), 29–42. Retrieved from http://www.itdl.org/Journal/May_11/May_11.pdf

Harden, R. M. (2005). A new vision for distance learning and continuing medical education. *Journal of Continuing Education in the Health Professions, 25*(1), 43–51. doi:10.1002/chp.8

Ho, K., Block, R., Gondocz, T., Laprise, R., Perrier, L., Ryan, D., . . . Wenghofer, E. (2004). Technology-enabled knowledge translation: Frameworks to promote research and practice. *Journal of Continuing Education in the Health Professions, 24*(2), 90–99.

Jakubec, S., Parboosingh, J., & Colvin, B. (2014). Introducing a multimedia course to enhance health professionals' skills to facilitate communities of practice. *Journal of Health Organization and Management, 28*(4), 477–494. doi:10.1108/jhom-09 -2012-0164

Mazzoleni, M., Maugeri, C., Rognoni, C., Cantoni A., & Imbriani, M. (2012). Is it worth investing in online continuous education for healthcare staff? *Studies in Health Technology Information, 180*, 939–943. doi:10.3233/978-I-61499-101-4-939

Parboosingh, J., Reed, V., Caldwell, J., & Bernstein, H. (2011). Enhancing practice improvement by facilitating practitioner interactivity: New roles for providers of continuing medical education. *Journal of Continuing Education in the Health Professions, 31*(2), 122–127. doi:10.1002/chp.20116

Pullen, D. (2013). Doctors online: Learning using an internet based content management system. *International Journal of Education & Development Using Information & Communication Technology, 9*(1), 50–63. Retrieved from http://ijedict.dec.uwi .edu/viewissue.php?id=34

Reed, V., Schifferdecker, K. E., & Turco, M. G. (2012). Motivating learning and assessing outcomes in continuing medical education using a personal learning plan. *Journal of Continuing Education in the Health Professions, 32*(4), 287–294. doi:10.1002/ chp.21158

Saba, F. (2016). Theories of distance education: Why they matter. *New Directions for Higher Education, 2016*(173), 21–30. doi:10.1002/he.20176

Vannieuwenborg, L., Goossens, M., De Lepeleire, J., & Schoenmakers, B. (2016). Continuing medical education for general practitioners: A practice format. *Postgraduate Medical Journal, 92*(1086), 217–222. doi:10.1136/postgradmedj-2015-133662

10

Technical Considerations to Support Learning Environments

Matthew J. Rietschel

INTRODUCTION

Nursing schools utilize technology in all aspects of academic and nonacademic activities. They use learning management systems (LMSs), content management systems, mobile learning, databases, social media, and virtual classrooms to create an online presence for learning to occur. Nursing education is using technology to supplement simulations, create virtual environments, engage in online games to mimic real-life situations, utilize electronic health records to simulate patient care, and review patient encounters for additional educational objectives. Nursing schools and licensing bodies are using computer-based assessments to determine if nursing students and registered nurses are prepared to move forward in their coursework and careers. These same practicing and student nurses are using technology to track and log millions of hours of professional development training or clinical hours as required. Finally, the use of Team platforms (e.g., Webex Teams, Microsoft Teams) that marry together a suite of tools has started to find a niche in nursing education, as well as research related to the nursing role. Although the focus is historically on the technology solutions itself, the necessary characteristics of the student, instructor/facilitator, and, more recently, senior leadership are as imperative to consider. These features are as important as the technology, as they drive the skilled, meaningful use of it. This importance can be demonstrated with a simple example: if two people buy the most expensive hammer available, and one has trained to be a master carpenter, but the other has not, who will be more capable of utilizing it to its full potential? This chapter examines the technologies and current trends, programmatic requirements, and student, faculty, and senior leadership traits to be successful in online learning environments and management systems used in nursing education.

USING TECHNOLOGY IN ONLINE LEARNING

Discussing the technologies in categorical terms and not by in-depth exploration of individual named software/hardware is necessary because of the breadth and speed at which the landscapes of the technology change. Therefore, this section discusses the categories of communication, Web 3.0, audio, video, creation tools, presentation tools, learning object repositories (LORs) in general, artificial intelligence (AI), and virtual reality (VR). The most important rule when incorporating technology is to ensure that it is appropriate to the learning objective and is not being used just because it is "cool" and new.

The 2018 New Media Consortium (NMC) *Horizon Report: Higher Education Edition* continues to show the trend of adaptive learning technologies (Adams Becker et al., 2018). Two technologies identified in the NMC 2013 report that span all of the previously outlined categories and this trend are mobile applications (apps) and tablet computing. In 2013, the NMC outlined the technologies with a high probability of adoption within 5 years (NMC & EDUCAUSE Learning Initiative, 2013). Everyone can agree that this prediction has proved to be quite true and that mobile devices and apps have found their way into almost every human endeavor. Tablet computer use is as ubiquitous as the use of personal mobile devices. Extensive tablet usage has become the standard, whether it be paying your bill tableside at a restaurant or a nurse charting at the bedside. Students who use tablets are showing positive learning outcomes, high levels of engagement, and knowledge retention (Patel & Burke-Gaffney, 2018). Mobile devices (i.e., smartphone and tablets) have become tools now used to further the key trends identified by the report for the short to long term, respectively: redesigning learning spaces, proliferation of open educational resources, and advancing learning experiences (Adams Becker et al., 2018).

Communication is the most important aspect of any course. The communication between the instructor and the class, the instructor and individual students, and student and student is vital to the online learning environment. Therefore, establishing communication avenues that are relevant to the course learning objectives, compatible with the technology infrastructure in place, and usable by the students is important. The three following examples are popular in the academic and corporate settings.

Web Conferencing

Schools are using web conferencing to conduct online information sessions for prospective students, faculty are using it to hold office hours, and research teams employ web conferencing to assemble members from far distances. Web conferencing surfaced in the late 1990s and is defined by PCMag.com (n.d.-b) as "a videoconferencing session via the Internet ... to interact with other participants, attendees use either a web application or an application downloaded into their client machines," and the definition is still applicable today. The main difference from 2013 is the ease and proliferation of how web conferencing occurs. In 2013, it was from a computer or dedicated system. It occurs today from mobile phones, tablets, interactive kiosks, and so forth. As in a live classroom, web conferencing allows faculty and students to meet and collaborate with easy, real-time conversation exchanges with immediate feedback, as well as greater opportunities for faculty to alter the pace of the instruction and to conduct student assessment (Schullo, Hilbelink, Venable, & Barron, 2007). Many web conferencing systems allow for shared web browsing, file transfer, common whiteboard space, and chat. Common conferencing solutions are Blackboard Collaborate (previously Wimba and Elluminate), Cisco's Webex, Citrix's GoToMeeting, and Adobe Connect. These tools are used in a vast array of applications from real-time monitoring of project-based learning in an IT (information technology) course in Spain (Marti et al., 2015) to eliciting probability distributions about uncertain model parameters from experts (Morris, Oakley, & Crowe, 2014).

Instant Messaging

Instant messaging (IM) is defined by PCMag.com (n.d.-a) as the exchange of text messages in real time (synchronous) between two or more people logged into a particular IM service. As with web conferencing, the definition has not changed since 2013, but the applicability and extent of use have grown exponentially, expanding the acronym to MIM—mobile instant messaging. Although IM has been around since the early 1990s and may seem like an outdated technology, it has evolved to have a place in online learning by employing the use of many input devices and exploiting the ease from which they can communicate with each other. Most platforms allow users to communicate via their computer, cell phone, or other mobile device, and some have expanded to allow features such as file sharing, audio messaging, and the use of avatars. IM can also be expanded into the use of a chat room, which allows multiple users to synchronously communicate in a common online area. MIM (especially WhatsApp—a multiplatform IM) has been shown to increase the educational affordances of students in higher education (Klein, da Silva Freitas Jun, da Silva, Barbosa, & Baldasso, 2018). The application of the technology is growing in use as a tool for follow-up with patients after medical procedures. For example, IM has been shown to be feasible and acceptable to communicate with patients during peritoneal dialysis treatment (Cao et al., 2018). Although IM and MIM can be used for sending short messages, in real time or delay, discussion boards in education still have a viable use for asynchronous discussion.

Discussion Boards

Discussion boards are also known as message boards, discussion groups, threaded discussions, bulletin boards, and online forums. They allow for an asynchronous conversation between two or more users with posted text or audio messages. The messages usually follow an outline or tree composition with the overall structure being a forum, a topical conversation thread, or a single message post. When a user responds to another user's post, the response is usually indented under the post to identify its relationship to other posts in the thread. A benefit of discussion boards over IM solutions is that the users do not need to be active in the environment at the same time, as messages archive on the board for later access. This benefit allows users to access messages on their schedule and provides them time to research and reflect to produce well-composed responses. Although most LMSs have a discussion board capability built into the platform, some common stand-alone discussion board solutions are Google Groups, phpBB, and vBulletin.

Web 2.0 and Web 3.0

Most people are familiar with the term Web 2.0, which was introduced in 2004, and it refers to technological improvements over what was

TABLE 10.1   Web 1.0/2.0/3.0 Summary

Crawl	Walk	Run
Web 1.0	**Web 2.0**	**Web 3.0**
Mostly Read-Only	Widely Read-Write	Portable & Personal
Company Focus	Community Focus	Individual Focus
Home Pages	Blogs/Wikis	Lifestreams/Waves
Owning Content	Sharing Content	Consolidating Content
Web Forms	Web Applications	Smart Applications
Directories	Tagging	User Behavior
Page Views	Cost Per Click	User Engagement
Banner Advertising	Interactive Advertising	Behavioral Advertising
Britannica Online	Wikipedia	The Semantic Web
HTML/Portals	XML/RSS	RDF/RDFS/OWL

Source: Fleerackers, T., & Meyvis, M. (2018). Web 1.0 vs Web 2.0 vs Web 3.0 vs Web 4.0 vs Web 5.0 – A bird's eye on the evolution and definition. Retrieved from https://flatworldbusiness.wordpress.com/flat-education/previously/web-1-0-vs-web-2-0-vs-web-3-0-a-bird-eye-on-the-definition

previously available to allow a different level of user interaction. The three most common Web 2.0 technologies are blogs, wikis, and social networking. Betrus (2012) reported that more than 70% of introductory technology courses for preservice teachers include the use of Web 2.0 technologies. Teachers report using Web 2.0 technologies to improve student learning, student-to-student interaction, student-to-instructor interaction, collaborative learning, and the sharing of content knowledge (Sadaf, Newby, & Ertmer, 2012). The term Web 2.0 has evolved into a new term, Web 3.0, which uses the knowledge accessible in 2.0 but adds the key feature of semantics (Table 10.1; Fleerackers & Meyvis, 2018).

By adding context to the vast amounts of data, the relevance of it increases and therefore intensifies its usefulness. For example, when a user searches for something on Facebook, the person's profile page and/or past history are used to present results that would be most relevant to that person. A simpler example would be to type *pizza* into a web browser. The results are for the history of pizza and shops within the local area. What if the same semantics could be applied to provide learners with information that was most pertinent to their learning style, needs, content area, and so on?

Audio and Video Media

The use of audio and video media is fast becoming as preferred by students as text-based materials. Distinct segments of students prefer audio material (such as podcasts) and videos to either digital or paper-based traditional learning materials (Robinson & Stubberud, 2012). One of the fastest-growing fields is the use of webcasting. Sonic Foundry is an example of a webcasting platform that allows for the capture, management, and delivery of webcasts for online training, conference presentations, executive briefings, and academic course sessions. More than 1,500 colleges and universities currently broadcast using Sonic Foundry's Mediasite webcasting solution to capture lectures (Sonic Foundry, 2018).

Creation and Presentation of Content

Faculty and students have the option to use many different types of tools for the creation and presentation of content. When deciding the best method to present or create material, it is important to remember that the technology used should be appropriate and related to the learning objective and not chosen because it is the newest technology. Some common, tried-and-true creation and presentation technologies are as follows:

- Google Docs: Allows users to create their work (documents, spreadsheets, surveys, etc.) online, work collectively, and easily share content with others (docs.google.com).
- YouTube: Allows users to upload original videos and to watch other users' videos on a wide array of topics (www.youtube.com).
- Prezi and SlideRocket: Web applications that have the benefit of storing the presentation online, easily incorporating graphical elements and enhanced visual effects to aid in audience engagement (www.sliderocket.com and prezi.com).
- Tiki-Toki: A web application used to create interactive timelines (www.tiki-toki.com).
- Visual.ly: A website with infographics and data visualizations. Users can either use the stored infographics on a variety of topics or create their own (visual.ly).

Learning Object Repository

LORs are databases that house learning objects (LOs) and provide easy access to individual resources such as simulations, multimedia, animations, videos, or a combination of several materials to form modules, lessons, and many other types of objects that are discipline specific. LOs are educational content that uses widely accepted specifications and standards that allow them to be searchable, interoperable, and reusable in different learning environments (Cechinel, Sicilia, Sánchez-Alonso, & García-Barriocanal, 2013; Margaryan & Littlejohn, 2008; McGreal, 2004). Frequently used LORs in academia are as follows:

- Kahn Academy (www.khanacademy.org)
- MERLOT (www.merlot.org)
- NOVA (science resources; www.pbs.org/wgbh/nova)
- TeacherTube (teachertube.com)
- University LORs (e.g., MIT Open Courseware, Texas A&M Digital Repository)
- State LORs (e.g., The Orange Grove, Florida's repository project)

A nursing-specific LOR is Quality and Safety Education for Nurses (QSEN). QSEN's (2013) goal is "preparing future nurses so that they will have the knowledge, skills, and attitudes (KSAs) necessary to continuously improve the quality and safety of the health care systems within which they work." This LOR is a central repository for information on competencies, teaching strategies, and faculty development.

Virtual Reality

VR allows a user to experience and manipulate an environment as if it were the real world. The digital environment is intended to simulate a person's presence in some part of it and still feel real. It was presented as a new development in technology to the congressional Subcommittee on Science, Technology, and Space in 1991 ("New Developments in Computer Technology: Virtual Reality," 1992) and has been used to train nurses since the mid-1990s (Dysart, 1996). There are various levels of VR, ranging from full immersion, in which all five senses are being stimulated, to more basic task-oriented environments. An example of a basic VR program would allow a nurse to virtually practice putting in an intravenous (IV) line on a digital arm with a digital needle, but by manipulating it with her actual hands. According to technopedia.com (2018), VR does not have a concrete definition, but follows some accepted guidelines: the environment comprises images that appear life-size according to the user's perspective, the system managing the VR is able to track the user's movements (i.e., eye, head, hand) and react to them, and the information should have both depth and breadth.

Artificial Intelligence

AI is defined in multiple ways; the easiest and most simplistic is that it is the intelligence of machines instead of people. The machine is able to work out an answer or solution by collecting and analyzing data. AI has been studied since the 1950s; Minsky (1952) sought to use AI in similar fashion to the human mind's ability to manipulate symbols. AI is all around us today and especially in healthcare. The learning or thinking happens when the machine is able to use its programming and what it has "learned" from previous experiences and apply it to influence its future actions. IBM Watson Health is the most well-known project in this field. It ingested millions of pages of academic literature and healthcare data to help providers make decisions by offering a series of suggestions with accompanying confidence interval for applicability. One fear of AI is that it will lessen what it means to be a human—the age-old apocalyptic scene from the future. Gregg (2018) states, "AI will not be able diminish the 'humanity' of human beings unless human communities allow it to do so" (p. 173). He states that only if society provides AI with those rights (i.e., human status, legal status), will it then have the capability to do so. The question of first developing AI that could have these rights is a discussion for another day, but AI in healthcare is here to stay and thrive.

MANAGEMENT SYSTEMS

Three main terms are used in describing management systems: learning, content, and course. The terms are used interchangeably in conversational vernacular when discussing management systems and education because all of the systems are usually accessed via the Internet and content can be loaded either through the same Internet access or by a local network connection. However, the interplay of these terms is not entirely accurate, and they draw from different historical contexts. If the terms are examined closely, they have very different meanings, although their meanings are usually equated to the context in which they are applied. The LMS software has its roots in corporate training and was originally designed for workplace learning environments. A course management system (CMS) is an online system that had its beginnings in academic settings. An example of how these systems are used is the delivery of academic courses for credit, professional development of faculty/staff, and training of students, and as an online space for organizations. A content management system (also CMS) is an environment that only stores content for access by other systems or users. This term is not to be confused with LMS or CMS, as it is a database for the storage of content items for access by other systems or directly by the user. Although LMSs offer some content storage options, content management systems offer more general and robust functions for managing content (Piotrowski, 2009). The content management system is not used to deliver education, but rather it is a repository with the ability to upload, manage, and download content artifacts (Catherall, 2008). Another acronym that is commonly used is LCMS, which can represent either learning content management systems or learning CMSs. These terms are used when systems are expanded to include characteristics of multiple systems. These various systems have grown over time, and the term LMS or learning management solution is currently used to define software that can manage, track, and deliver educational programs or courses. As the terms LMS and CMS are used synonymously, this definition can be applied to both terms.

The three most popular LMSs (Pappas, 2014), based on total customers, active users, and online presence, are as follows:

- *Moodle*: "A software package for producing Internet-based courses and websites. It is a global development project designed to support a social constructionist framework of education" (Moodle, 2013).
- *Edmodo*: "A free and safe way for students and teachers to connect and collaborate" that "helps connect all learners with the people and resources needed to reach their full potential" (Edmodo, 2013).
- *Blackboard*: "Blackboard helps clients enrich all aspects of the education experience by engaging and assessing learners, making their daily lives more convenient and secure, and keeping them informed and aware of the most important information" (Blackboard, 2013).

Even though the terms ultimately have different meanings, the meanings are usually equated to the context in which they are applied. Therefore, to understand the capabilities of a specific system, one must look past the term used to describe it and more closely at the characteristics of the systems to determine the best solution for their expected use. As this book is focused on the development of online learning environments, the term used in this chapter to describe the systems will be LMSs.

LMSs have core functionality that allows them to perform the necessary functions for learners, faculty, and administrators. These functions

TABLE 10.2   Technical Specifications and Key Features of LMSs

Key Feature	Administrator/Instructor	Student/Learner
Core Learning Tools	• Content management • Support for multiple content types • Communication • Collaborative learning tools • Content standardization • Social media integration	• Communication • Collaborative learning tools • Personalization • Ability to create learning pathways • Intelligent content suggestions • Gamification tools
Assessment	• System reporting • Reporting across multiple courses • Customizable	• Progress dashboard • Feedback tools • Badging • Rubrics • Portfolios
Technical	• Open or closed source • Integration with other systems (e.g., SIS, API) • Permission levels • Single sign-on (SSO) authentication	• Ease of help • System support services • System and web browser needed
Accessibility	• Multiplatform accessibility • Accessibility compliance/ compatibility	• Multiplatform accessibility • Intuitive up-to-date interface
Usability	• Infrastructure to maintain and support • Managing users	• Learning curve to utilize • Ability to work offline

API, application programming interface; SIS, student information system.

fall into the four categories of communication, administration, productivity tools, and course delivery tools. These four core function areas and the characteristics related to hardware/software and licensing information are all important features to understand to choose a system and use it to its full potential. There are websites and services designed to compare the different features; examples are Edutools.com, which is focused on academic systems, and a report from FindtheBest (2013), which compares systems used for corporate learning. Administrators and/or instructors should consider the key features of an LMS when determining which system will be a good fit for their needs. The most significant features and tools are outlined by category in Table 10.2.

The decision on what LMS to use rarely falls upon faculty. There are some exceptions, usually large institutions that have multiple systems so that faculty will have the opportunity to choose which system they will use to teach a course or training. The ideal method for selecting the LMS for an institution is by a consortium that comprises the informational technology office (technology infrastructure), faculty (needs of the learners and content of the courses), the program directors (curriculum and reporting needs), and the financial group (budget). The process should be a slow one and incorporate all of the LMS feature needs and the requirements of the institution. The faculty and program directors should focus on the learner and support tools as outlined in Box 10.1. The informational technology office and financial group will focus on the technical specifications, which are outlined in Table 10.3.

Along with the learner, support, and technical features to consider, other systems on campus should weigh in on the decision as well. The ideal process for selection of an LMS is to conduct a needs assessment on all of the areas outlined previously, decide the most important learner and support tools, and then match the best technical specifications to meet the academic, infrastructure, and financial needs. Although the LMS is the heart of the technology used in teaching an online course, it is not the only technology available to instructors and students. Other technologies can be integrated into the LMS or used as a stand-alone to supplement the online learning process.

STUDENT REQUIREMENTS

A student must have certain skills and have access to specific items to be a successful online learner. Nursing students have been found to lack knowledge of basic computer software, email and communication skills, and college-specific software related to traditional, hybrid, and online courses (Edwards & O'Connor, 2011). Some of the requirements to be an online student are basic, such as access to a computer and the Internet. These basic needs are communicated by the institution to the student as technical requirements. The technical requirements are specific to the needs of the school, the LMS, and other technologies the student requires during the pursuit of a degree. An example of the technical requirements for different nursing programs is usually found in the new student or technology section of the school's website. Other skills such as a student's readiness to be an online learner and ability to use the LMS are

---

BOX 10.1

Technology Knowledge and Abilities

The competent instructor is knowledgeable about the technologies used in the virtual classroom (online classroom) and can make effective use of those technologies.

Access: The competent instructor ...

- Has access to the required technical equipment and software for the given medium and the course
- Owns or has easy access to necessary technical equipment and software including a computer, a reliable Internet connection, and other equipment such as video editing that might be required by the given course and content

Technical Proficiencies: The competent instructor ...

- Is knowledgeable about and has the ability to use computer programs that are typically required in online education to improve learning/teaching, personal productivity, and information management
- Has an understanding of various commonly used web-browsing software programs
- Is proficient in the chosen course management system
- Can modify content within the system as necessary
- Can manage all student activities within the learning management system (LMS)
- Has clear abilities within the primary communication channels of the LMS
- Has the ability to use word processing software including the ability to compose documents using accessibility software as required
- Has the ability to use and manage asynchronous and synchronous communication programs
- Has proficiency managing a computer operating system to maintain security updates, virus scanning software, and other software updates as necessary for the course

Source: Adapted from Varvel, V. E., Jr. (2007). Master online teacher competencies. *Online Journal of Distance Learning Administration, 10*(1), 1–47.

---

not easily measured, but are equally important. Basic and advanced online assessment tools help students determine if online learning is a good fit for them and if they have the skills to be successful. A basic free quiz to determine if distance learning is appropriate for a student is offered by The University of Iowa and can be found at distance.uiowa.edu/courses/are-you-ready-online. Smartmeasure.com is a more robust

TABLE 10.3   Comparison of LMS Technical Specifications

Fee Type	Free Commercial

Source Code
  Availability
	Open source
	All the files that make up the system are free for modifying,
	  which allows customizing the system in the necessary way
	Proprietary
	Do not provide the source code

Licensing Models	Per number of registered/enrolled users Per number of concurrently connected users Per license validity period Per number of courses

Installation Type	Hosted (software as a service)
	Installed on the vendor's hardware at a vendor controlled
	  location
	Own
	Installed on the local site or network and provides complete
	  control of all processes

Business Orientation	eCommerce Educational institutions Corporate training Government structures

Programming Language	Multiple languages
	Important due to impact on technology infrastructure,
	  future programming costs, and other systems desired to
	  integrate

Platform	Stand-alone solution Integrated solution

Integration	Open source
	Provides the widest range of integration possibilities
	Documented application programming interface, or API
	  (software development kit, or SDK)
	Provides the use of one application to be used by another
	  application
	Integration via bridges
	Special plug-ins that allow the integration of different types
	  of applications

LMS, learning management system.
Source: Adapted from Joomla. (2013). *Learning management system comparison.* Retrieved from
http://www.joomlalms.com/compare

online assessment tool that is a "124-item assessment which measures a learner's readiness for succeeding in an online and/or technology rich learning program" and "indicates the degree to which an individual student possesses attributes, skills and knowledge that contribute to success in learning" (SmartMeasure, 2018). The site measures components in seven areas:

- Individual attributes: motivation, procrastination, willingness to ask for help, and so forth
- Life factors
- Learning styles
- Technical competency
- Technical knowledge
- On-screen reading rate and recall
- Typing speed and accuracy

Students should also know how they learn best or their learning style. This information will help them to determine if distance learning is a good fit for them and what resources they should seek. There are free online learning style inventories, such as the one offered at EducationPlanner.org (www.educationplanner.org/students/self-assessments/learning-styles -quiz.shtml, 2018).

INSTRUCTOR REQUIREMENTS

An online instructor needs to have a different set of competencies than an instructor who only teaches in the traditional classroom. The most important of these competencies is to know that instructors must seek assistance in developing, designing, and planning for the technology used in their course. Although many faculty are experts in the content and are talented teachers, "faculty members cannot be expected to know intuitively how to design and deliver an effective online course … seasoned faculty members have not been exposed to techniques and methods needed to make online work successful" (Palloff & Pratt, 2001, p. 23). The instructor must be able to adapt both the teaching style and the content to create the most advantageous learning environment for students. Nguyen, Zierler, and Nguyen (2011) surveyed 193 faculty members from nursing schools in the western United States and found that while 66% of faculty reported they were competent with distance-learning tools, 69% reported a need for additional training. Some of the required information is the same regardless of whether the instruction happens online or in a traditional classroom. Both modalities require the instructor to know the most up-to-date content, who the learners are, and how the course relates to the overall program. But the online instructor needs to have additional information and must overcome barriers specific to the online environment (Table 10.3). Institutions, colleges, programs, and courses will have specific technology requirements of the instructor; therefore, it is important to think about necessary competencies in generalizable terms and not specific skills (e.g., expert in the use of Microsoft Office version 2010). Varvel (2007) composed a list of instructor competencies that is relevant and applicable to all online instructors.

LEADERSHIP REQUIREMENTS

The scale of implementing and supporting technology requires innovation with senior leadership and champions at each supporting level. The student and instructor responsibilities have been covered previously, but the role of the senior leadership is equally important. In 2004, Marcus completed a literature review of the management of distance education and deemed that there was not enough current evidence to create a "concrete definition" of a distance education leader (Marcus, 2004). Although a concrete definition may never be agreed upon by all, the traits and skills of an effective distance education leader are well described in the present-day literature. The first item that needs to be evident is that leadership is willing to be innovative, flexible, and responsive (Salyers et al., 2012). This need may cause anxiety for some leadership that values a highly structured environment and process. Therefore, Salyers et al. (2012) state that finding a balance between "creativity, responsiveness, and stability" is necessary to sustain a distance education program. Joshi and Shahi (2015) found that administrators are poised to be innovative as shown by their readiness to develop competencies in conducting a qualitative research approach via distance e-learning. This shows that administrators understand the benefits that online learning can bring to different and new initiatives. Nworie, Haughton, and Oprandi (2012) examined 191 distance education position announcements between 1997 and 2010 to investigate the qualities and qualifications sought by higher education. Their investigation concluded that the needs of this position are quite broad and require a graduate level degree as well as varied experiences in academia, administration, strategic planning, operations, and leadership (Nworie et al., 2012). Leadership must not only possess the wherewithal to make bold decisions, but must also have the broad range of skills to do it effectively.

SUMMARY

LMSs continue to be hubs on which institutions base their online learning, but a variety of accompaniments are being added to enhance the student experience and expand the instructor's toolbox for education. These accompaniments provide improved communication, increased collaboration, and the creation and distribution of high-quality audio/video LOs. With the ever-expanding market for online education and technology, it is important to reinforce the true reason behind using any technology—to support the learner, instructor, and learning objectives at all levels. In order for the technology used to reach its maximum potential, instructors and students need to embrace the necessary competencies, be creative, and always be open to a new learning opportunity. Although the role of online education is proven to be effective, the digital technologies are not enough to transform the very nature of teaching and learning in higher education (Henderson, Selwyn, & Aston, 2017); therefore, the technology, the student, the instructor, the senior leadership, and infrastructure all have important roles in the achievement of this transformation.

REFERENCES

Adams Becker, S., Brown, M., Dahlstrom, E., Davis, A., DePaul, K., Diaz, V., & Pomerantz, J. (2018). *NMC horizon report: 2018 higher education edition.* Louisville, CO: EDUCAUSE.

Betrus, A. (2012). Historical evolution of instructional technology in teacher education programs: A ten-year update. *Techtrends: Linking Research & Practice to Improve Learning, 56*(5), 42–45. doi:10.1007/s11528-012-0597-x

Blackboard. (2013). *About blackboard.* Retrieved from http://www.blackboard.com/About-Bb

Catherall, P. (2008). Learning systems in post-statutory education. *Policy Futures in Education, 6*(1), 97–108. doi:10.2304/pfie.2008.6.1.97

Cao, F., Li, L., Lin, M., Lin, Q., Ruan, Y., & Hong, F. (2018). Application of instant messaging software in the follow-up of patients using peritoneal dialysis, a randomised controlled trial. *Journal of Clinical Nursing, 27*(15/16), 3001–3007. doi:10.1111/jocn.14487

Cechinel, C., Sicilia, M.-Á., Sánchez-Alonso, S., & García-Barriocanal, E. (2013). Evaluating collaborative filtering recommendations inside large learning object repositories. *Information Processing & Management, 49*(1), 34–50. doi:10.1016/j.ipm.2012.07.004

Dysart, J. (1996). VR simulator to train student nurses... virtual reality. *Nursing & Allied Healthweek, 1*(12), 19. Retrieved from http://survey.hshsl.umaryland.edu/?url=http://search.ebscohost.com/login.aspx?direct=true&db=rzh&AN=107340266&site=eds-live

Edmodo. (2013). *Features*. Retrieved from http://www.edmodo.com/about

Edwards, J., & O'Connor, P. A. (2011). Improving technological competency in nursing students: The passport project. *Journal of Educators Online, 8*(2), 1–20. doi:10.9743/JEO.2011.2.2

FindTheBest. (2013). *Compare learning management systems*. Retrieved from http://lms.findthebest.com

Fleerackers, T., & Meyvis, M. (2018). *Web 1.0 vs Web 2.0 vs Web 3.0 vs Web 4.0 vs Web 5.0 – A bird's eye on the evolution and definition*. Retrieved from https://flatworldbusiness.wordpress.com/flat-education/previously/web-1-0-vs-web-2-0-vs-web-3-0-a-bird-eye-on-the-definition

Gregg, B. (2018). The coming political: Challenges of artificial intelligence. *Digital Culture & Society, 4*(1), 157–180. doi:10.14361/dcs-2018-0110

Henderson, M., Selwyn, N., & Aston, R. (2017). What works and why? Student perceptions of 'useful' digital technology in university teaching and learning. *Studies in Higher Education, 42*(8), 1567–1579. doi:10.1080/03075079.2015.1007946

Joomla. (2013). *Learning management system comparison*. Retrieved from http://www.joomlalms.com/compare

Joshi, S., & Shahi, M. (2015). Deliberations of nursing academics towards distance education. *Journal of Institute of Medicine, 37*(1), 55–60.

Klein, A. Z., da Silva Freitas Jun, J. C., da Silva, J. V. V. M. M., Barbosa, J. L. V., & Baldasso, L. (2018). The educational affordances of mobile instant messaging (MIM): Results of Whatsapp® used in higher education. *International Journal of Distance Education Technologies, 16*(2), 51–64. doi:10.4018/IJDET.2018040104

Marcus, S. (2004). Leadership in distance education: Is it a unique type of leadership—A literature review. *Online Journal of Distance Learning Administration, 7*(1). Retrieved from https://www.westga.edu/~distance/ojdla/spring71/marcus71.html

Margaryan, A., & Littlejohn, A. (2008). Repositories and communities at cross-purposes: Issues in sharing and reuse of digital learning resources. *Journal of Computer Assisted Learning, 24*(4), 333–347. doi:10.1111/j.1365-2729.2007.00267.x

Marti, E., Gil, D., Gurguí, A., Hernández-Sabaté, A., Rocarías, J., & Poveda, F. (2015). PBL on line: A proposal for the organization, part-time monitoring and assessment of PBL group activities. *Journal of Technology and Science Education, 5*(2), 87–96. Retrieved from http://survey.hshsl.umaryland.edu/?url=http://search.ebscohost.com/login.aspx?direct=true&db=eric&AN=EJ1135487&site=eds-live

McGreal, R. (Ed.). (2004). *Online education using learning objects. Open and Distance Learning Series*. London, England: Routledge/Falmer.

Minsky, M. (1952). *A neural-analogue calculator based upon a probability model of reinforcement*. Cambridge, MA: Harvard University Psychological Laboratories.

Moodle. (2013). *About moodle*. Retrieved from http://docs.moodle.org/24/en/About_Moodle

Morris, D. E., Oakley, J. E., & Crowe, J. A. (2014). A web-based tool for eliciting probability distributions from experts. *Environmental Modelling & Software, 52*, 1–4. doi:10.1016/j.envsoft.2013.10.010

New developments in computer technology: Virtual reality, Hearing before the Subcommittee on Science, Technology, and Space of the Committee on Commerce, Science, and Transportation, Senate, 102 Cong, 1st sess, May 8, 1991. (1992). Washington, DC:

Government Printing Office. Retrieved from http://survey.hshsl.umaryland
.edu/?url=http://search.ebscohost.com/login.aspx?direct=true&db=edsgpr&
AN=edsgpr.000371413&site=eds-live

New Media Consortium and EDUCAUSE Learning Initiative. (2013). *NMC horizon report: 2013 higher education edition.* Retrieved from https://www.nmc.org/nmc-horizon

Nguyen, D. N., Zierler, B., & Nguyen, H. Q. (2011). A survey of nursing faculty needs for training in use of new technologies for education and practice. *Journal of Nursing Education, 50*(4), 181–189. doi:10.3928/01484834-20101130-06

Nworie, J., Haughton, N., & Oprandi, S. (2012). Leadership in distance education: Qualities and qualifications sought by higher education institutions. *American Journal of Distance Education, 26*(3), 180–199. doi:10.1080/08923647.2012.696396

Palloff, R., & Pratt, K. (2001). *Lessons from the cyberspace classroom: The realities of online teaching.* San Francisco, CA: Jossey-Bass.

Pappas, C. (2014). *The 20 best learning management systems (2018 update).* Retrieved from https://elearningindustry.com/the-20-best-learning-management-systems

Patel, S., & Burke-Gaffney, A. (2018). The value of mobile tablet computers (iPads) in the undergraduate medical curriculum. *Advances in Medical Education and Practice, 9,* 567–570. Retrieved from http://survey.hshsl.umaryland.edu/?url=http://search.ebscohost.com/login.aspx?direct=true&db=edsdoj&AN=edsdoj.9f2be174b2db41aabfb229f4574adf94&site=eds-live

PCMag.com. (n.d.-a). Definition of instant messaging. Retrieved from https://www.pcmag.com/encyclopedia/term/45045/instant-messaging

PCMag.com. (n.d.-b). Definition of web conferencing. Retrieved from https://www.pcmag.com/encyclopedia/term/54287/web-conferencing

Piotrowski, M. (2009). Document-oriented e-learning components (Doctoral dissertation). Magdeburg, Germany: Otto von Guericke Universität. Retrieved from https://files.eric.ed.gov/fulltext/ED533734.pdf

Quality and Safety Education for Nurses. (2013). *About QSEN.* Retrieved from http://qsen.org/about-qsen

Robinson, S., & Stubberud, H. (2012). Student preferences for educational materials: Old meets new. *Academy of Educational Leadership Journal, 16,* 99–109.

Sadaf, A., Newby, T. J., & Ertmer, P. A. (2012). Exploring factors that predict preservice teachers' intentions to use web 2.0 technologies using decomposed theory of planned behavior. *Journal of Research on Technology in Education, 45*(2), 171–196. doi:10.1080/15391523.2012.10782602

Salyers, V., Tarlier, D., Van Pelt, L., Bailles, J., Beaveridge, J. S., Lapadat, C., & Robertson-Laxton, L. (2012). Growing an innovative faculty-driven management team in a distance-delivery NP education program: Thinking outside the box to meet the nursing education and health needs of northern British Columbia, Canada. *Journal of the American Academy of Nurse Practitioners, 24*(9), 528–535. doi:10.1111/j.1745-7599.2012.00725.x

Schullo, S., Hilbelink, A., Venable, M., & Barron, A. E. (2007). Selecting a virtual classroom system: Elluminate Live vs. Macromedia Breeze (Adobe Acrobat Connect Professional). *JOLT, 3.* Retrieved from http://jolt.merlot.org/vol3no4/hilbelink.htm

SmartMeasure. (2018). *SmartMeasure about.* Retrieved from http://www.smarter services.com/solutions/smartermeasure/about

Sonic Foundry. (2018). *Why Mediasite by Sonic Foundry.* Retrieved from http://www .sonicfoundry.com

Technopedia. (2018). *Virtual reality.* Retrieved from https://www.techopedia.com/ definition/4784/virtual-reality

Varvel, V. E., Jr. (2007). Master online teacher competencies. *Online Journal of Distance Learning Administration, 10*(1), 1–47. Retrieved from https://www.westga .edu/~distance/ojdla/spring101/varvel101.htm

11

Course Management Methods

Cheryl A. Fisher

INTRODUCTION

Many instructors are expected to deliver high-quality instruction to people who would otherwise not be able to participate in higher education. This presents an exciting and challenging opportunity for collaborative learning and is affecting the way traditional classes are taught. In 2017, according to the Babson Survey Research Group's Higher Education Reports, the growth of distance enrollments has been relentless (Allen, Seaman, & Seaman, 2018). Distance student enrollment has increased for the 14th straight year with enrollment up 5.6% exceeding gains seen over the past 3 years. Now at least 31.6% of all students take at least one distance education course (a total of 6,359,121 students).

Distance students are fairly evenly split between those who take both distance and nondistance courses (3,356,041 students) and those who take exclusively distance courses (3,003,080). Nearly 6.7 million students participated in distance learning, and nearly one third of all students are taking at least one online course (Allen et al., 2018). Managing an online course can have many similarities to managing a face-to-face course but will differ in complexity with the use of existing and emergent technologies and geography. However, it is through the use of this rapid expansion and application of technology that the online learning environment is becoming a richer and sometimes preferred place to learn.

Facilitating learning at a distance requires faculty to take some new approaches to managing the teaching and learning process. The faculty role in the online classroom requires greater attention to detail, structure, and monitoring of student activity. According to Vitale (2010), effective online faculty is becoming critical to deal with the nursing shortage, and faculty must learn to manage a new set of variables that determines the extent to which their courses are effective. In this chapter, the role of the instructor in planning, organizing, and managing the online learning environment, along with the expectations of the student, is discussed.

FACULTY ROLE

The role of the instructor shifts from the traditional classroom "sage on the stage" to the "guide on the side." Although these might be overused phrases, there is a lot of truth to them when applied to the instructor role shift that takes place when teaching online. In a traditional setting, the instructor feeds information to students in a lecture or PowerPoint slide presentation format, creating a teacher-centered environment. This method of teaching has long been used in educational settings and has come to be what most students expect. In a distance learning role, the instructor focuses on discussing and reviewing materials presented through video and audio technologies, assigned readings, and interactive group activities. The faculty role is that of a content expert who guides or facilitates student learning through direction to resources and stimulation of discussion, thereby creating a student-centered environment. A trained facilitator is important to the success of an online program, and the prospects can be overwhelming to faculty new to online teaching. The facilitator's training, personality, professionalism, and knowledge of the content become important factors influencing the online classroom.

Faculty training for teaching online may differ significantly from face-to-face instruction. Currently, there is no single approach, and many institutions are using a combination of training and mentoring. Ninety-four percent of institutions with online offerings report that they have training or mentoring programs for their online faculty. The most common training approaches for online faculty are internally run training and informal mentoring. Some smaller institutions report looking to outside institutions for their training needs.

According to the Illinois Online Network (ION, 2018), the responsibilities and pressures on instructors require faculty to look at teaching students in a new way. Some feel the pressure of a classroom that is open

24 hours a day with adult learners who might require additional support owing to their already busy lives. Some responsibilities include:

- Planning and organizing the course
- Creating a collaborative atmosphere
- Constructing open-ended, thought-provoking questions
- Providing direction and leadership
- Sequence and pace
- Giving feedback
- Netiquette
- Special considerations
- Faculty
- Students

To perform the preceding responsibilities, successful online faculty should have some basic background knowledge and preparation to teach online. The ION (2018) identifies that the online instructor should have a broad base of life experiences in addition to academic credentials in the subject matter. This will enable the instructor to actively participate with students and guide their constructive thinking. Other skills required to be successful include:

- Be open, concerned, flexible, and sincere so one can compensate for the lack of physical presence.
- Feel comfortable communicating in writing.
- Believe that learning can occur in facilitated online learning environments.
- Believe that the online learning process includes learning information that can be used today and that requires critical thinking.
- Be supportive of the development of critical thinking.
- Have the appropriate credentials to teach the subject.
- Be well trained in teaching and learning online.

Teaching in a technology-rich environment is complex and therefore requires a broader set of skills and competencies from the faculty facilitators to ensure success. A study conducted by Bigatel, Ragan, Kennan, May, and Redmond (2012) identified competencies and teaching tasks aimed at providing faculty with professional development in critical competencies to ensure online teaching success. These competencies focused on the areas of active learning and engaging with students as appropriate, administration and leadership, active teaching and providing prompt helpful feedback, use of multimedia appropriate for learning activities, classroom decorum to help students resolve potential conflicts, technological competence, and policy enforcement. These competencies closely mirror but expand on the seven principles of effective teaching identified by Chickering and Ehrman (1996).

PLANNING AND ORGANIZING

When planning and organizing an online course, the instructor must look at the overall course in terms of objectives, outcomes, assessment, and evaluation. The planning should include the criteria discussed in the reconceptualization chapter of this book (Chapter 6, Reconceptualizing the Online Learning Environment). The instructor should keep in mind that it is in this beginning phase of course development that an instructional designer and an information technology expert should be consulted for best practices.

The curriculum of an online program must be designed especially for the collaborative nature of online learning. Course content should be organized in modules with clear deadlines for the assigned work in each section. These concise lectures should be compensated with open-ended remarks and discussion questions that will elicit comments and provide the students opportunities to contribute a variety of viewpoints. The curriculum should focus on applying knowledge utilizing real-world examples and fostering critical thinking skills within the opportunities of exchanging ideas. Instructors should give clear and simple assignments with clear instructions.

COLLABORATION

Once the course has been planned and organized, the instructor is ready to launch the course. It is now the instructor's responsibility to create a collaborative atmosphere. To create this environment, the students should encounter a friendly, welcoming message as they first enter the online course. Using an "ice breaker" such as requesting a short biography and a photo as the initial assignment will give students something to which they can respond. The instructor can post his or her bio as an introduction and then ask the students to present theirs in a similar format. This is not only a way of introducing oneself to the class but also a way for the instructor to gain information about students that can be used later in class discussions. The students often find that they have similar backgrounds or professional interests, which then allows them to begin developing a sense of community through realization of shared goals and shared expectations of the course. By asking the learners to contribute their goals and expectations, the instructor is able to determine if his or her approach to the course will correspond more closely to the needs of the learners.

Students should be encouraged to respond to each other's postings. The best way to teach students how to post meaningful statements is for the instructor to model how they should respond. Modeling a short but welcoming response does this best. Not only does this enable students to begin opening up to each other, but it begins to create a safe space in which they can interact. The posting of an introduction is the first step in revealing who one is to the others in the class, and it is critical that students feel acknowledged so they can continue to do that safely throughout the duration of the course. This is the first point of connection—the point where these important relationships begin to develop.

DEVELOPING DISCUSSION QUESTIONS

Developing or creating open-ended questions is the primary method for stimulating discussion, assessing student learning, and providing for interactivity among the learners. More and more evidence is emerging about the value of interaction between faculty and students to promote effective teaching. The discussion questions should be based on the desired learning outcomes and can vary in number based on instructor preference. The discussion questions should be open ended, thought provoking, and relevant to student learning. Then, the instructor as well as the students must learn the art of expansive questions to keep the discussion going. This allows the responsibility for facilitation of discussion to be shared among all participants. And finally, students should be encouraged to provide constructive feedback to one another throughout the course. Rather than being at the forefront of the discussion, the instructor is an equal player, acting as a gentle guide. The sharing of this responsibility among the participants is one way instructors can stretch their facilitative skills.

The discussion questions should be developed in such a way that there is no right or wrong answer. They serve to stimulate thinking and are a means by which the instructor can assess students' learning and understanding of the issues. The instructor needs to model this form of questioning so that students can learn to answer questions in a substantive manner, provide an example, cite a resource, and end with an expansive question of their own for their peers. This allows for the discussion to progress to a higher level as questions are answered and expanded upon by students pursuing the issue. The instructor's role is to closely monitor the discussion and to jump in with another question, thereby expanding the level of thinking beyond the original question. A poor or minimal response to a question could indicate that student thinking has not been stimulated and that the learners have not been compelled or inspired to respond. Commenting on discussion questions by asking students for more information or by sharing some aspects of their professional expertise can help to engage students and facilitate online discussions.

Some examples of the behaviors that faculty must exhibit to meet the competency of active learning include encouraging student interactivity by assigning them to team projects and groups for project purposes and encouraging shared knowledge by providing opportunities for hands-on practice so that students can apply learned knowledge to the real world, for example, with problem-solving activities and peer-to-peer assessment. These tasks can promote active learning and are skills required by faculty to promote learning.

DIRECTION AND LEADERSHIP

Providing direction and leadership in an online course should begin before the students enter the classroom. The syllabus or a separate document on how to run the course provides clear directions for students about the following aspects of the course:

- General information
- Contact information
- Textbooks or other course materials
- Course requirements
- Where to start
- How I plan to run this course
- Class schedule, parts of the classroom
- Group work and expectations
- Technical support

- Grading
- Student responsibility

General course information to include in the syllabus should include course start and end dates, project due dates, and midterm and final exam dates. Time off for spring break or other breaks related to holidays or official closing of the university should also be included on the course calendar. Contact information is important for students to have easy access to faculty. Often, it is helpful to put a primary and a secondary email address, work and home phone numbers (optional), and the best times to make contact. Times of contact are important, especially when students are working shifts and faculty may be located in a different time zone. Required texts and supporting documents should be available to students before class begins or at least during the first week of class. Students should have the ability to order books from either the bookstore or another online book service such as Amazon. Other recommended texts should be listed in case students are interested in purchasing these as well.

Course requirements help students know in advance what they will need to do and what faculty has identified as requirements to complete this course, for example, view lecture material, complete assigned readings, participate in team exercises, complete assignments, and take midterm and final examinations. Listing requirements ahead of time will help students organize their approach to the course and will provide clarity of course requirements.

"Where to start" and "How I plan to run this course" documentations are opportunities to help students begin. In a face-to-face course, this is the housekeeping session that takes place on the first day of class. When directing students where to start, it is critical to have students attend either a face-to-face or an online orientation. It is in this orientation that they will be instructed to obtain a password for the course and begin to learn basic navigation of the courseware if this is their first experience with online learning. Once students are inside the online course, they should be directed to read the course information carefully. This should include the syllabus and all supporting documents that will be used to run the course.

The course schedule can be placed in a calendar and should include important dates that students should note, for example, weekly lectures and when discussion questions will be posted. This schedule will help students develop some structure for their learning and help them to juggle their workload. Let them know when quizzes will be posted, and again take the opportunity to highlight due dates of midterms, final exams, and papers. The instructor should make sure that students know how to access grades. One lesson for faculty that cannot be overstated is that you cannot be too redundant in the online environment. The more places a student can find important dates, the better. The main parts of the classroom should also be clearly delineated. If using courseware such as Blackboard or Moodle, the left menu bar is a good place to start designing the online classroom. For example:

Announcements: Frequent communications and important dates to remember should be posted here.

Course Information: This section should contain documents such as the syllabus, quizzes, sample of an American Psychological Association–formatted paper (or whatever style guide is required), instructions on submitting assignments, and other pertinent documents.

Faculty Information: This section should contain contact information (as identified previously) as well as other information that might be useful while students are enrolled in your course.

Assignments: This section should contain instructions for individual assignments and the grading criteria.

Course Documents: This section houses course lectures, course objectives, readings, and supplemental web links for each lecture of the course. This is the primary location for the course content.

Student Tools: This is where the digital drop box, student grades, calendar, and other tools are located.

By identifying the parts of the online classroom, orientation information is restated, and a text document is provided for reference. Once this document is written, it is highly reusable except for dates or changes that have taken place in the course. Technical support contact information should also be provided in the form of hours of availability, phone numbers, and email. Although this information is provided, invariably technical questions will show up in the discussion area of the classroom. Posting a message thread for technical questions will often allow students to answer each other's questions and keep the questions separate from the course content of the main classroom.

Grading information should also be clearly delineated in terms of (1) methods of evaluation (i.e., class exercises, assignments, papers, rubrics, and exams) and (2) criteria for the final grade. For example:

- Participation 10%
- Team Exercises 30%
- Midterm Exam 30%
- Final Exam 30%
- Total 100%

Just as in face-to-face classes, students need to know the weight of graded assignments. They should also know what percentage or point value is required for letter grades. This is also a good place to include the policy on late assignments (regarding point reduction) or incomplete grades and information about the university's policy on academic integrity.

One aspect of ensuring quality and academic integrity is finding ways to document student identity as related to course assignments and testing. In short, faculty need to be sure that individuals receiving course credit are, indeed, the individuals who do the work. Institutions have a variety of ways to achieve identity security in the context of a meaningful assessment. The choices that an institution has will depend on the institutional resources, the type of assessment appropriate for measuring achievement of the learning objectives, and the number of students who need to be served. Although high-tech methodologies exist for secure identification, such as retinal scanning or facial, voice, or fingerprint identification, institutions may not be ready to invest in these technologies. Another alternative is proctored testing centers or web-based testing software. This software requires a user name and password and can provide a different test each time the user logs in. Faculty should be familiar with the capabilities of the course management system, or they can consult with technical support to determine best options.

SEQUENCE AND PACE

The sequence and pace of providing lectures and assignments can be left to the instructor's discretion. Some instructors prefer to post lectures, assignments, and discussion questions on a weekly basis. This controls the pace of the course and does not allow the students to work ahead. This model would most closely replicate the sequence and pace of a face-to-face classroom. Some instructors like to guide the online classroom discussion using this strategy. Another option would be to release course content by units or modules. Using this strategy, the instructor would still want to control the discussion by posting discussion questions regularly within the block of time designated for a particular unit. A third strategy for sequencing the release of course content would be to give the student the entire course at the beginning of class. Students will be required to participate according to the instructor's instructions. This strategy allows students to work ahead in their reading, writing, and group work, but it also allows the instructor to control the collaborative learning in the main discussion area of the classroom. Some instructors have found it useful to put start and stop dates on discussions. For example, if a particular discussion thread is only going to be open for 2 weeks, the instructor should post start and stop dates at the beginning of the message thread so that students know when to move on to the next topic.

FEEDBACK

Feedback is one of the most critical activities that instructors need to be aware of in online learning because of the lack of face-to-face interaction. Feedback goes beyond confirmation of correct answers. Feedback is necessary for students to develop new understandings and to facilitate learning. Students need much more support and feedback in the online environment than in a traditional course to compensate for the lack of face-to-face interaction (ION, 2018). It is necessary for instructors to respond to students in a timely manner (usually within 24–48 hours) in order for students to feel encouraged to participate and to continue to participate at a high level. Online students need extra reinforcement and verification of their performance. Positive feedback, constructive feedback, and tone are all areas that instructors need to be aware of and sensitive to when responding to students. For example, proposing an alternative viewpoint might be interpreted by a student as an incorrect statement on the student's part as opposed to just an expansion of ideas. While maintaining a positive and encouraging tone and keeping things light with humor and emoticons (www.netlingo.com/smileys.php), the instructor can still maintain a professional atmosphere in the class environment.

Most instructors know that communicating with students can positively influence learning and can be done using feedback techniques. Because improvement in learning is more likely to occur following both written and oral critiques of student work, it is important to provide more than just a number or letter grade on student assignments. Written critiques or telephone conversations can be provided to students for more in-depth explanations of grades, but it is more likely this will occur by email. The following characteristics should be considered in providing personal feedback to students:

- Multidimensional (covers content, presentation, and grammar)
- Nonevaluative (provides objective information)
- Supportive (offers information that will allow the learner to see areas for improvement)
- Receiver controlled (allows the learner to accept or reject the information)
- Timely (provided as soon as possible after the intended work)
- Specific (precisely describes observations and recommendations)

The instructor should be sure to provide information at the beginning of class so that students know what is expected of them and what will be standard for evaluation and feedback. Instructor feedback should be clear, thorough, consistent, equitable, and professional. As students require regular and constructive feedback from faculty, they will appreciate comments that indicate the instructor has tailored remarks for that particular individual.

NETIQUETTE

Netiquette, or Internet etiquette, is a type of guideline for posting and sending messages in the online classroom. Netiquette not only covers rules of behavior but also provides guidelines for ensuring smooth interaction in the online environment. Shea (2011) outlined core rules of netiquette that every online student and instructor should follow:

- Remember the human (never forget there is really a person behind the keystrokes).
- Adhere to the same standards of behavior online that you follow in real life (in other words, be ethical).

- Know where you are in cyberspace (i.e., main discussion area, group forum).
- Respect each other's time and bandwidth (post appropriate messages).
- Make yourself look good online (check grammar and spelling).
- Share expert knowledge (help answer others' questions).
- Help keep tempers under control (do not respond to irate postings).
- Respect other people's privacy (do not read others' private email).
- Do not abuse your power.
- Be forgiving of other people's mistakes (you were once new to the online environment as well).

The core rules of netiquette were designed to help students who are new to the Internet to make friends instead of enemies. The instructor can post a link to these basic rules to help students understand the basic expectations of behavior online.

SPECIAL CONSIDERATIONS

Diversity and Americans with disabilities are global issues facing us daily and occur as well in the online environment. As these issues are sensitive to many people, instructors should consider human equity issues seriously. Diversity consists of two dimensions: primary and secondary.

Primary dimensions are those characteristics that everyone is born with and that are visible and easy to identify. They include age, gender, race, ethnicity, and other physical characteristics.

Secondary dimensions are differences or characteristics that we acquire or change throughout our lives. These include work experience, income, marital status, religious beliefs, and education. These dimensions shape everyone we encounter in school, the workplace, and social settings (Center for Research on Education, Diversity, and Excellence, n.d.).

Government agencies, corporations, and educational institutions are now recognizing the necessity of valuing diversity to remain competitive and effective. As a facilitator, one needs to eliminate stereotypes and become more educated about different groups. This way, one is less likely to generalize. Suggestions for doing this might include:

- Becoming aware of the stereotypes you hold
- Determining the source of the stereotype and how it was formed

- Expanding your knowledge about other groups and cultures
- Expanding your experiences with other groups and cultures

KEY POINTS OF AMERICANS
WITH DISABILITIES ACT

The Americans with Disabilities Act Home Page identifies security and testing issues in distance learning. They direct universities to make their distance learning classes accessible to qualified individuals with a disability, just as they are required to do for traditional courses. Specifically, Title 42 U.S.C. section 12132 states: "Subject to the provisions of this subchapter, no qualified individual with a disability shall, by reason of such disability, be excluded from participation in or be denied the benefits of the services, programs, or activities of a public entity, or be subjected to discrimination by any such entity" (Sec. 202). For nonpublic institutions, 42 U.S.C. section 12182 provides: "No individual shall be discriminated against on the basis of disability in the full and equal enjoyment of goods, services, privileges, advantages or accommodations of an entity" (Sec. 301). These provisions protect and ensure Americans with disabilities equal access to online education and all information provided to the general public.

As universities and faculty expand their distance education offerings, they are finding that they must include the virtual equivalents of wheelchair ramps when building their online classrooms. They must accommodate, for instance, the student who is unable to see navigational graphics on a webpage due to blindness and the student who cannot listen to a streaming audio lecture because of deafness. In fact, many students with disabilities find that most website technological extravaganzas are more of a burden than an aid.

For the most part, distance education students with disabilities can already get the equipment they need to make up for their impairments. Blind students can use software that reads online text aloud or produces a Braille message for the students to follow. Students who cannot move their arms easily can use adaptive equipment to manipulate the computer with other parts of their bodies. But some common features of the Internet make navigation difficult for people with certain disabilities. Text reading programs, for instance, are unable to recognize graphics. The problem is easily avoided if the programs can pick up and read aloud alternate texts that are placed behind the graphics, but not every website provides those texts. Sites with frames and tables (two commonly used features of webpage design) tend to confuse those programs, which often read from left to right, ignoring the layout. An important issue is for universities to determine exactly what the law requires.

As an online facilitator, considerations for students with disabilities need to be taken on an individual basis. For example, if you know a student who has a particular disability, you will need to take into account accommodations that may be necessary for the particular problem. It should be determined from the beginning exactly what the student's limitations are and what devices the student is using, if any, for example, text telephones (TTY phones), screen readers, or voice recognition software. Allowing more time for test taking may be necessary, or allowance for leniency on spelling if you know a student is using voice recognition software. Check with your institution for policy regarding disabilities. If you are using audio files, for example, be sure to include a text version of the same information. If you are including web references, be sure to check their format (amount of graphics, use of frames) for accommodating screen readers. The bottom line is that everyone should have equal access to information.

FACULTY DEVELOPMENT

Effective training for online faculty is imperative in order for quality instruction to be delivered. This training may be 1 to 2 weeks in length and may be paid or unpaid (Bristol & Zerwekh, 2011). As it becomes more evident what quality online instruction looks like, it will be necessary to incorporate training on the competencies associated with quality instruction into a comprehensive faculty training program (Bigatel et al., 2012). Faculty preparation for teaching online measurably improves learning effectiveness and satisfaction (Moore, 1993). The ION's *Making the Virtual Classroom a Reality* and the *Master Online Teacher certification* programs provide the skills, understanding, and knowledge needed to be a successful online teacher. The ION's website (www.ion.uillinois.edu/resources/) provides institutions with tools and resources for developing their own programs for faculty training. Faculty training is becoming so critical that even iTunes (itunes.apple.com/us/itunes-u/faculty-development-for-online/id421439101) and YouTube (www.youtube.com/watch?v=m3H7PbkndOk) are posting faculty development snippets or brief training videos on developing an online course, fostering student interaction, distance learning and Web 2.0, and other topics.

THE SUCCESSFUL DISTANCE STUDENT

The student role in a distance course also changes significantly from a face-to-face classroom. Students must be more responsible for their own learning, must be able to communicate through writing, and must possess certain characteristics that will ensure their ability to participate successfully in an online program. There is greater emphasis on identifying one's own learning needs and making plans to achieve learning objectives. In other words, online learning takes self-direction and discipline on the part of the distance student. The ION describes what the profile of a successful online student looks like (ION, 2018). Prior to becoming an online student, the individual must have some basic knowledge of information technology to participate in a distance course. Gilbert (2001) suggests that students start by asking:

- What is online learning, and what is it like?
- Where can I find it, and is it for me?
- What works in an online environment?
- What criteria make a good candidate for online learning?
- What are the advantages or disadvantages?
- How do I choose an online learning provider?
- How do I pick a curriculum?
- How can I get information about sources?
- What makes for a good distance program?
- Where do I start?
- How can I succeed?
- How can I manage the tools and equipment?

When designing distance learning academic programs, the basic characteristics of students should be considered. Their ages, interests, skill levels, academic preparedness, and career goals, for example, all should be considered. Much of the literature suggests that older students and adults are the primary participants in distance programs. In the United States, typical adult distance learning students are between the ages of 25 and 50. Many online learners are adult students with family and job responsibilities who require the flexibility of online learning to advance in their jobs or to earn their degrees. However, as more and more students become exposed to the online learning model, the traditional profile is changing.

In your online course, you may want to include reference links to resources and tips for your students to use to help them be more successful online learners. Many universities have information on their home page with tips for success in online courses. Clearly outlining expectations and characteristics of a successful online student can help students determine if the online environment will be a productive learning environment for them. Questionnaires for prospective students to use to assess whether they are good candidates for online learning can often be found on the university home page.

SUMMARY

With the shift in faculty role finally realized, online course management involves a breadth of considerations including student orientation, the importance of discussion, instructor feedback, and evaluation methodologies. The importance of collaboration is one of the most critical areas facilitating learning with shared responsibility between the faculty and the students. Structuring a course for ease of navigation should be as user friendly as possible so as not to detract from the course content. Awareness of diversity and disabilities is critical in management of online courses as student needs may not be obvious. Faculty preparation for putting courses online should be addressed with professional training and peer feedback to ensure that best practices and current evidence support the course structure.

REFERENCES

Allen, E., Seaman, J., & Seaman, J.; Babson Survey Research Group. (2018). *Higher education reports.* Retrieved from https://www.onlinelearningsurvey.com/high ered.html

Americans with Disabilities Act of 1990, Pub. L. No. 101-336, 104 Stat. 328 (1990).

Bigatel, P., Ragan, L., Kennan, S., May, J., & Redmond, B. (2012). Identification of competencies for online teaching success. *Journal of Asynchronous Learning Networks,* 16(1), 59–77. doi:10.24059/olj.v16i1.215

Bristol, T. J., & Zerwekh, J. (2011). *Essentials of e-learning for nurse educators.* Philadelphia, PA: F. A. Davis.

Center for Research on Education, Diversity, and Excellence. (n.d.). Retrieved from http://www.cal.org/crede

Chickering, A., & Ehrman, S. (1996). *Implementing the seven principles: Technology as lever.* Retrieved from http://www.tltgroup.org/programs/seven

Gilbert, S. (2001). *How to be a successful online student.* New York, NY: McGraw-Hill.

Illinois Online Network. (2018). Retrieved from http://www.ion.uillinois.edu/resources/tutorials/overview/elements.asp#The%20Facilitato%20r

Moore, M. (1993). Theory of transactional distance. In D. Keegan (Ed.), *Theoretical principles of distance education* (pp. 22–38). New York, NY: Routledge.

Shea, V. (2011). *Net etiquette*. Retrieved from http://www.albion.com/netiquette/introduction.html

Vitale, A. T. (2010). Faculty development and mentorship using selected online asynchronous teaching strategies. *Journal of Continuing Education in Nursing, 41*(12), 549–556. doi:10.3928/00220124-20100802-02

12

Assessment and Evaluation of Online Learning

Carol A. O'Neil and Cheryl A. Fisher

INTRODUCTION

The new directions and emerging guiding structures of online education require changes in the methods of student assessment and program evaluation. Assessing the learner involves gathering data to identify needs, ability, and progress. Assessment is student oriented, and the goals are to place, promote, graduate, and/or retain students. Evaluation is a judgment made by comparing a behavior to a standard. Evaluation is the measurement of a behavior and the comparison of that behavior to a predetermined expectation.

ASSESSMENT, EVALUATION, AND PEDAGOGY

Evolving methods of teaching and learning influence assessment and evaluation. Learning modalities, such as massive open online courses (MOOCs), certificates, and competency-based education (CBE), require a change in the processes of assessment and evaluation.

Regardless of emerging assessment and evaluation strategies, pedagogical theory forms the basic framework for the design of a learning experience. The learning experience is a process that starts with the purpose for the learning opportunity. Objectives flow from the purpose. The learning strategies logically flow from objectives, and the evaluation also appropriately flows from the objectives. For example, if the learning objective is to state five signs and symptoms of congestive heart failure, the evaluation should measure whether the learner can state them. To determine if the student has achieved this objective, the student may find a question on a test to name five signs and symptoms.

A traditional evaluation design does not include the use of technology as a teaching and learning tool. Technology influences the course before it is offered, while it is being offered, and at the end of the course.

Precourse student assessment and remediation built into the design of the learning experiences assess technology skills and allow the learner to practice the skills so the student has direct access to the learning material when the course starts. For example, the online student should have the computer skills needed to negotiate the online course, should have the needed resources (i.e., course entry information such as username and password), and should know how to navigate through the course. If the student does not have these basic skills, the student will have to spend time learning navigational skills instead of the course material. These precourse assessments should provide data about the student's readiness to be successful in online courses. Gaps in knowledge and skills provide information for developing a prescriptive plan that will guide the learner to resources needed to be successful online. The prescriptive plan is written and individualized for each student and includes activities and outcomes that focus on the skills that will ensure success online. Some examples are knowing how to download files, navigating the web, receiving and sending email, sending attachments, and basic typing skills.

When developing learning material online, the learning material should be peer reviewed before the course starts. Peer review is a process in which a designated reviewer uses established criteria to review a course. Information gathered from the review allows the course developers to make corrections before students log on to the course. A peer review is crucial for newly developed courses, because there may be links that do not work, spelling and grammatical errors, or even exam dates in the syllabus that are not the same as the dates on a calendar. The purpose of a peer review is to enhance the quality of learning for the student. The reviewer has a "fresh set of eyes" that can detect errors so they can be corrected before the learners arrive.

A peer review while the course is live is also recommended. During the course, servers can crash, and hard drives can go down. For example, during one semester, a student assignment included gathering secondary data about a community. Data about the behavioral indicators of a community, such as smoking, obesity, prenatal care, and so forth, were located on a server managed by the state health department. About a week before starting content on the community assessment module, the state health department took down the information. The faculty checked the links to this website before the course started, and therefore, they did not know that the link was not working when the students started the assignment. Monitoring the course during implementation might have enabled them to find and fix this problem earlier. Early in the course, the faculty can ask students to email them with anything that looks like a course issue as soon as it becomes apparent. Give students permission to ask "dumb" questions like "Should the syllabus icon link to the syllabus?" Faculty needs information to correct "glitches." Aside from technical issues, there could be learner issues. Students may be struggling with understanding the content or staying on schedule with assignments. Conflicts between students may develop, or there could be hurt feelings because someone typed a negatively perceived comment. A quick response to technical and student issues while the course is running prevents further (and usually more chaotic) repercussions.

At the end of the course, faculty, learners, and instructional designers use tools that focus on gathering data that are particular to online courses to evaluate the course. Evaluation provides information that contributes to making decisions about the course. There are two types of evaluation: formative and summative. Formative evaluations provide information for revising the instruction, and summative evaluations provide data about the continued use of the instruction.

A process of recognizing faculty members for their contributions to and successes with online learning enhances motivation. Faculty who teach online should request that content and technology experts "sit in" on their courses as guests to provide feedback. This feedback can be included in a tenure and promotion package, to promote recognition of scholarship of teaching and learning online, and to provide visibility for online courses, especially to faculty who do not teach online.

In summary, assessing learners' skills and abilities is an essential component in online learning. Learners need feedback during the course while they are constructing new knowledge, and they need grades assigned at the end of the course. The course needs reviewing before it goes live, during implementation, and when it is completed. Therefore, traditional assessment and evaluation models need modifications to accommodate learning online.

MODEL FOR ASSESSING AND EVALUATING ONLINE TEACHING AND LEARNING

The authors of this chapter developed a model that incorporates the foundations of assessment and evaluation of online learning. Assessment and evaluation are activities that are part of the course design. They should be appropriate measures of the goals and objectives of the learning experience. The activities provide information to make judgments about student learning and course effectiveness. Comprehensive activities include information about the feasibility of student success online, the progress of the student through the course, student achievement of the course objectives at the end of the course, the effectiveness of the course design, the effectiveness of the course during implementation, and the outcomes of the course. The proposed model focuses on student learning and course evaluations separately.

Assessment focuses on the student, and evaluation focuses on the course. Assessment and evaluation are components of the course design and are visible throughout the course from before the beginning of the course until after the course ends.

Assessment is the identification of student needs and progress throughout the learning experience. The purpose of precourse assessments is to identify the needs of the student before the course begins. During the course, the focus is on the student's progress. The faculty monitors the student throughout the course and gives feedback about the process of constructing knowledge. Assessing the learner at the end of the course involves graded activities. Evaluation focuses on the course itself. Precourse evaluation includes peer review of the course before it starts. Formative evaluation determines how the course is operating, and summative evaluation involves evaluation of the course after it is completed.

The model for assessing and evaluating learning online is shown in Figure 12.1. The relatedness of the three phases for student assessment and three phases of course evaluation from the start of the course to the end is depicted.

During each phase, evidence is gathered and analyzed, and decisions result. During the continuous assessment phase, students receive feedback. The end student assessment is the measure of individual achievement based on the student's ability to meet objectives, and a decision to pass or fail is determined.

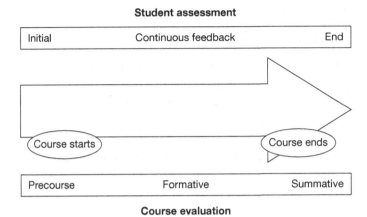

FIGURE 12.1   The model for assessing and evaluating learning online.

STUDENT INITIAL ASSESSMENT

The following list includes some suggestions for faculty to use when conducting an initial student assessment prior to participating in an online course:

- Initial letter of assessment about the student as a learner
- Placement exams
- Students develop personal webpages
- Electronic meeting
- Computer skills exercise
- Pretests
- Scavenger hunt to assess navigation skills (develop a scavenger hunt list and posting of announcements; ask students to find the items and email the answers to the instructor)
- Learning style surveys
- Readiness surveys

Continuous Feedback

Continuous student feedback occurs at any time during the course. The purpose of continuous feedback is to determine if the student is learning from the course material presented. It is important for the faculty to know if the course material is clear and logical. Obtaining this information prior to the end of the course enables the instructor to make changes. Some of these techniques include:

- Journaling, writing marathons, keeping diaries. These techniques assess attitude and satisfaction (affective objectives)
- Creating written logs about experiences and reflections
- Concept mapping: connective key concepts
- Giving midsemester assessment
- Estimating student time ranges for each assignment plus interaction
- Giving feedback
- Having 3-minute "things I do not understand about" sessions
- Assigning a weekly new idea
- Debating
- Asking students to answer the question "What was the fuzziest point?"
- Assigning reaction paper
- Assigning worksheets
- Giving nongraded quizzes
- Using simulations
- Assigning crossword puzzles
- Tracking attendance
- Allowing peer questions to other students
- Encouraging participation in discussion board
- Assigning homework
- Questioning
- Assigning case studies, which are detailed accounts of a client, family, group (e.g., pregnant teens), or community

COMPLETING A STUDENT ASSESSMENT

At the end of a course, a determination is made about students meeting the course learning objectives. The following list identifies some methods:

- Quizzes
- Compositions, essays, and papers
- Projects (individual or group): project summaries, webpage presentations
- Analysis of articles

- Examinations: Exams can be multiple choice and/or essay type
- Portfolios (efolios)
- Student presentations
- Peer evaluation
- Final interviews
- Rubrics

PRECOURSE EVALUATION

Precourse evaluations guide faculty in determining if the course is ready for launching. Ideally, an external, objective reviewer should review the course for content and for instructional design. The peer reviewer should then continue to observe the course for interaction approximately 2 weeks into the course and again at midterm. The reviewer provides constructive feedback to the instructor for changes. Preevaluation activities can include:

- Peer review of content
- Peer review of design

Formative Evaluation

Formative evaluation throughout the course allows the faculty to determine if course delivery, structure, or instructional design needs revising. Some suggestions for formative evaluation are:

- "Pulse Check": Ask students on a regular basis, maybe every 4 weeks or three times during the semester, to post or email their "pulse"— where they are and how they are doing in the course and what improvements or changes they think should be made
- Discussion summaries every other week about course content and issues
- Midsemester survey
- Verbal feedback to specific questions
- Summative evaluation: Summative evaluation obtains information for revising the course and evaluating. This evaluation provides feedback to the faculty to revise the course and to evaluate the faculty
- Student evaluation of the course
- Student evaluation of faculty
- Faculty evaluation of the course

RESOURCES

Several resources are available that focus on assessment and evaluation. Faculty Focus Special Report (2011) provides an overview of assessment. Refer to the sections titled "Educational Assessment and Online Learning." The information presented supplements the model described in this chapter.

The Illinois Online Network (2018) offers topics on student assessment and course evaluation, such as homework, rubrics, and cheating. The information provided gives definition to the phases presented in this chapter.

Cornell University Center for Teaching Innovation (n.d.) provides information about measuring student learning, peer assessment, feedback, rubrics, and more. This information provides more depth to the content of this chapter.

A resource for evaluating online courses is Quality Matters. Quality Matters is a toolkit and a process for certifying quality of online courses (Quality Matters, 2018). There are 8 general standards—course overview and introduction, learning objectives, assessment and measurement, instructional material, learning activities and learner interaction, course technology, learner support, and accessibility and usability (Quality Matters, 2018)—and 42 specific standards included in the review of a course.

The Online Learning Consortium (OLC, n.d.) suggests an evaluation design called the OLC Quality Scorecard that includes categories (administrative support, technology support, course development, instructional design, course structure, teaching and learning, social and student engagement, faculty support, student support, and evaluation and assessment). Quality is expressed by points, and a maximum of 225 points can be scored.

UW-LaCrosse offers Online Course Evaluation Guidelines for validating course quality. The guidelines consist of five categories (course overview and information and content, learning objectives and learner engagement, learner support and accessibility, interaction/presence, and assessment and feedback) that are ways to design, deliver, and improve quality of online courses (UW-LaCrosse Online Course Evaluation Guidelines, n.d.).

Rubrics are sets of standards used to assign grades and give students feedback about their performance. Rubrics can use descriptions or commentaries on achievement, such as excellent, good, fair, or poor, or they can be numerical. Rubistar (2008) is an online resource to guide developing rubrics.

SUMMARY

A model has been developed that can be used to assess student learning and evaluate the learning environment. It incorporates the foundations of assessment and evaluation and online learning. Student assessment determines needs before the course starts, measures progress during the course, and assesses attainment of goals at the end of the course. The course should be peer evaluated before it is released to students. Frequent evaluation of the course during implementation allows for the identification of problems and issues that can be remedied. Evaluating the course at the end provides data to revise the course and data to redesign.

REFERENCES

Cornell University Center for Teaching Innovation. (n.d.). *Assessment and evaluation.* Retrieved from https://teaching.cornell.edu/teaching-resources/assessment-evaluation

Faculty Focus Special Report. (2011). *Educational assessment: Designing a system for more meaningful results.* Retrieved from https://www.facultyfocus.com/free-reports/educational-assessment-designing-a-system-for-more-meaningful-results

Illinois Online Network. (2018). *Assessment and evaluation topics.* Retrieved from www.ion.uillinois.edu/resources/tutorials/assessment/index.asp

Online Learning Consortium. (n.d.). *OLC Scorecard for the administration of online programs.* Retrieved from https://onlinelearningconsortium.org/consult/olc-quality-scorecard-administration-online-programs

Quality Matters. (2018). *Maryland online.* Retrieved from https://www.qualitymatters.org/qa-resources/rubric-standards

Rubistar. (2008). *What is a rubric?* Retrieved from http://rubistar.4teachers.org/index.php?screen=WhatIs&module=Rubistar

UW-LaCrosse Online Course Evaluation Guidelines. (n.d.). Retrieved from https://www.uwlax.edu/globalassets/offices-services/catl/guidelines.pdf

13

The Changing Role of the Nurse Educator

Carol A. O'Neil and Cheryl A. Fisher

INTRODUCTION

Shifts in the workforce have historically resulted in shifts in education. Notable shifts, called education revolutions, are the expansion of high-school education and the development of associate degree education. An intent of both of these programs was to prepare learners for the workforce. The advent of computers and technology influences the workforce in that machines rather than people perform tasks. Job elimination results, and training for new skills for new jobs expands. Automation leads to a rapid change in demand for knowledge and skill that high-school and college education can no longer provide. A student chooses a major, and the skills needed for a job in that major will most likely change before the student graduates. Thus, higher education is in a new revolution of training for a lifetime of employable skills. Using artificial intelligence (AI) will change the way we currently perform in our jobs, and the first step in knowing how to change education to accommodate future needs is achieved by "big picture thinking" that is multidimensional and multidisciplinary (West & Allen, 2018). The potential workforce in need of training and retraining includes undereducated workers, unemployed workers, workers whose jobs are shifting due to automation, and gig economy workers who are independent, self-employed contractors. Training and retraining focus on job skills, and current sources are federal retraining and employer retraining.

It is no longer the case that high school prepares learners for college work. College does not provide the job skills required, as automation and the economy changes. There will be new employment positions and gaps in current positions that employees will need to train for by developing new skills. The movement entails shorter, skills-specific training to prepare for changes in economy, jobs, and the workforce. This is the new face of lifelong learning.

The role of higher education will shift from an emphasis on job skills to building skills to prepare for the jobs of the future (Desire2Learn, 2018), some of which are unknown today. The important skills are critical thinking, collaboration, design, visual display of information, and independent thinking (West & Allen, 2018).

The National Association of Colleges and Employers (NACE, 2018) defines career readiness as possessing competencies that are needed for a successful transition from education to practice:

- Critical thinking/problem-solving
- Oral and written communications
- Teamwork and collaboration
- Digital technology
- Leadership
- Professionalism and work ethics
- Career management
- Global and intercultural fluency

THE FUTURE LEARNING ENVIRONMENT

The characteristics of the learning environment amenable for learning these skills are described in Planning for the Future of Online Learning (Desire2Learn, 2018) as lifelong, accessible, digital, practical, contextualized, relevant, aligned with outcomes, and personalized in that the content is student centered and aligned with goals, interests, and experience. Respondents to a study by Evans (2018) found that nurse educators want to teach in a stimulating and flexible work environment and are encouraged about influencing the profession in a time of change.

THE TECHNOLOGY

Matthew Lynch (2018) describes expected changes in technology that impact online learning. One is mobile learning, which will enhance access to online learning environments. Mobile learning, also called m-Learning, provides access to resources and support on a mobile device so learners have anytime and anywhere access to information. The second is a teaching strategy called project-based learning in which students use technology to interact with peers to resolve problems. The problems are authentic and provide the learners with knowledge about the problem and with communication skills to work with peers. The third change is the use of learning analytics and visualization software that will provide feedback to learners about their learning process. Learning analytics is the gathering and the organizing of data to generate conclusions. Visualization is the display of the conclusions into a format that the learner will understand and use. An example is gathering data that support a learner as kinesthetic. The conclusion shows the learners their learning style and the learning strategies that will best accommodate their style. The next change is a redesign in online classrooms that allows for smart classrooms for learning in real time and for guest speakers. The fifth change is a movement to blended learning environments that will allow for online and classroom learning. Adaptive learning technology will employ software that adapts to the learners' learning needs and styles. The learning environment begins with basic information and requests an assessment response from the learner. The response leads to the next set of content. An example is a language package that begins with basic vocabulary and questions about knowledge of the vocabulary. A response of mastery will lead to higher level learning content. Technology provides enhanced teaching and learning strategies that will influence the learning process.

THE ROLE OF THE FACULTY EDUCATOR

A majority of faculty members have taught online classes. Eighty-nine percent report involvement in developing these courses, and 25% secured this help from an instructional designer (Jaschik & Lederman, 2018). Most of the faculty members who collaborated with instructional designers described their experience as positive, and about 70% reported an improvement in the quality of their course because the instructional designer suggested the technology that contributed to student learning. Legon and Garrett (2018) suggest that when the institution of higher education requires instructional design support, there is an increase in student-to-student interaction in online courses.

The role of the faculty member is to collaborate with an instructional designer to build these learning environments. Roles should be clear but shared. The faculty member is the content expert, and the instructional designer will ensure that the content delivered is in the most appropriate way for learning to occur via the technology. They should understand each other's role and build meaningful collaboration (Milosch, 2018).

THE EXPECTATIONS OF THE FUTURE FACULTY EDUCATOR

The educator is required to have a vast set of skills that support the design of transitioning course content into the online learning environment. These skills include the following:

- Develop, implement, and evaluate active learning strategies that support active learning.
- Focus on alignment in educational endeavors.
- Collaborate with an instructional designer.
- Develop flexible learning environments.
- Include technical and supportive skills content.
- And most important, have fun.

Another pertinent factor regarding the future of nursing education is the continuing trend in the shortage of nursing faculty. Nurse educators are aging and retiring, and too few younger nurses are coming in to replace them (Evans, 2013). In 2014, nursing programs denied entry to 68,938 applicants because of the faculty shortage (National League for Nursing, 2015). Although this number is down from previous years, it remains critical to continue to build the nursing workforce, as the population in general continues to age and the need for qualified nurses will continue to increase. One way of doing this is by increasing access to education through online programs with nursing faculty trained with these skills.

A final consideration and one of the most important is that of the changing landscape based on societal shifts, generational differences, and the impact of technology. The Institute of Medicine (IOM), now called the National Academies of Sciences, Engineering, and Medicine (Lippincott Solutions, 2018), have called on nurses to take a bigger role in America's healthcare system to help meet its increasingly complex and changing demands. The committee addressed nurses' roles, settings, and educational levels in planning for the future. The key messages included the following conditions:

- Nurses should practice to the full extent of their education and training.
- Nurses should achieve higher levels of education and training through an improved education system that promotes seamless academic progression.
- Nurses should be full partners, with physicians and other healthcare professionals, in redesigning healthcare in the United States.
- Effective workforce planning and policy making require better data collection and information infrastructure.

Currently, increased numbers of nurses are now practicing with doctoral degrees, nurse practitioners are practicing with fewer barriers, increased numbers of nurses are serving on boards or other governing bodies, and the diversity of the nursing workforce is showing growth (Lippincott Solutions, 2018). With these positive trends in nursing as a profession, it appears that nurse educators are on target to support the evolving requirements of our future healthcare professionals. With the support from nursing education and evolving requirements, nurse educators are in a position to create flexible learning environments as an alternative to traditional learning. The expansion and adoption of online nursing programs that are emerging are using creative technological innovations that will support the future needs of the nursing workforce.

SUMMARY

Changes in technology and automation influence the way nurse educators teach nursing. The educational trend is moving toward lifelong learning so knowledge and skills can be updated as changes in the work environment occur. Institutions of higher education prepare students for lifelong learning by including soft skills, such as critical thinking and communication, in the curriculum. Flexible and creative learning environments enhance accessibility of learning. The role of faculty members is to use technology in teaching to create authentic, problem-based learning strategies. Including the instructional designer in designing courses that include the technology-based strategies is a priority.

REFERENCES

Desire2Learn. (2018). *Planning for the future of online learning.* Retrieved from https://d12v9rtnomnebu.cloudfront.net/paychek/Planning_for_the_future_of_online _learning.pdf

Evans, J. D. (2013). Factors influencing recruitment and retention of nurse educators reported by current nurse faculty. *Journal of Professional Nursing, 29*(1), 11–20. doi:10.1016/j.profnurs.2012.04.012

Evans, J. D. (2018). Why we became nurse educators: Findings from a nationwide survey of current nurse educators. *Nursing Education Perspectives, 39*(2), 61–65. doi:10.1097/01.NEP.0000000000000278

Jaschik, S., & Lederman, D. (2018). *The 2018 inside higher ed survey of faculty attitudes on technology.* Retrieved from https://www.insidehighered.com/system/files/media/IHE_2018_Survey_Faculty_Technology.pdf

Legon, R., & Garrett, R. (2018). *The changing landscape of online education (CHLOE) 2: A deeper dive.* Retrieved from https://encoura.org/project/chloe-2/

Lippincott Solutions. (2018). *Update of the future of nursing report—Are we there yet?* [Blog post]. Retrieved from http://lippincottsolutions.lww.com/blog.entry.html/2018/02/13/update_on_futureof-q5jh.html

Lynch, M. (2018). *What is the future of online learning in higher education?* Retrieved from https://www.thetechedvocate.org/future-online-learning-higher-education

Milosch, T. (2018, January 17). *Building a collaborative instructor-instructional designer relationship.* Retrieved from https://www.insidehighered.com/digital-learning/views/2018/01/17/building-collaborative-instructor-instructional-designer

National Association of Colleges and Employers. (2018). *Career readiness defined.* Retrieved from http://www.naceweb.org/career-readiness/competencies/career-readiness-defined

National League for Nursing. (2015). *Findings from the 2014 NLN biennial survey of schools of nursing academic year 2013-2014* [Executive summary]. Retrieved from http://www.nln.org/docs/default-source/newsroom/nursing-education-statistics/2014-survey-of-schools---executive-summary.pdf?sfvrsn=2

West, D. M., & Allen, J. R. (2018, April 24). *How artificial intelligence is transforming the world.* Retrieved from https://www.brookings.edu/research/how-artificial-intelligence-is-transforming-the-world

Index

active learning, 9, 21, 112, 170
  in blended courses, 71, 73, 79
  online, 23, 141–142, 144
  by PBL scenarios, 54–55. *See also*
    problem-based learning (PBL)
  process, 23, 28, 36
  strategies, 79
  techniques, 8
adaptive learning, 47, 57–58, 120, 169
adult learners
  busy lives of, 110, 141, 153
  characteristics of, 21–22, 28
  social interaction and learning
    outcomes, 25–26
adult learning, 21–22, 28
  in NPD, 92, 99–100, 104
  principles, 55, 56, 92, 99–100, 104,
    114
affective networks, 39, 40
AI. *See* artificial intelligence (AI)
alternative learning, 6–7, 16–17.
    See also competency-
    based education (CBE);
    microcredentials/
    microcredentialing; open
    educational resources (OER);
    stackable degrees
Americans with Disabilities Act, 151
artificial intelligence (AI), 15–16, 120,
    126, 167
assessment and evaluation, 157–165

formative evaluation, 159, 160, 161,
    163
model for, 160–161
peer review, 158, 160
precourse evaluation, 160, 163
precourse student assessment, 158
prescriptive plan, 158
resources for, 164–165
student assessment, 161–163. *See
    also* feedback, continuous
  completion of, 162–163
  initial, 161
summative evaluation, 159, 160,
    161, 163
asynchronous communication, 4, 7,
    8, 48, 51, 60, 72, 77, 80, 95, 98,
    122, 130
automation, 3–4, 14–16, 167–168, 171

badges/badging, 7, 59, 60, 61, 128.
    See also microcredentials/
    microcredentialing
  digital, 59, 60, 97
behaviorism, 24–25, 28
blended courses, 1, 6, 66
  clarification of course delivery
    methods, 74, 77
  classroom-based sessions, 71–72
  community building, 71–72, 78
  delivery formats, 70, 72, 73–77,
    80–82

student-to-student interactions, 51, 169

Health Insurance Portability and Accountability Act (HIPAA), 97
higher education, 11–18
and career development, 13–14
and employment opportunities, 14–16
enrollment in institutions, 11–12
Higher Education Act, The (1965), 14
technology, effect on, 12–13, 15, 17–18. *See also* m-learning (mobile learning)
tuition, impact on, 12
HIPAA. *See* Health Insurance Portability and Accountability Act (HIPAA)
Horizon Report, The, 12, 120
hybrid courses. *See* blended courses
hybrid learning. *See* blended learning

ID. *See* instructional design (ID)
IM. *See* instant messaging (IM)
"Implementing the Seven Principles: Technology as Lever," 7–9
instant messaging (IM), 121–122
instructional design (ID), 37, 39, 43, 48, 54, 65, 163, 164, 169
instructional designers, 18, 50, 55, 100, 142, 159, 169–170, 171
Instructional Enhancement Initiative, 3–4
interactions, interpersonal, 7–9, 21–22. *See also* communication
asynchronous (delayed), 4, 7, 8, 48, 51, 60, 72, 77, 80, 95, 98, 122, 130
discussion, 4, 23, 25, 48, 49, 59, 94, 122, 143–144. *See also* discussion boards

face-to-face. *See* face-to-face interaction
instructor-to-student, 50
introduction session, 71, 72, 77–78, 142–143
learner-to-content, 48–49, 50–51
learner-to-instructor, 48, 50, 55
learner-to-learner, 48–49, 51
m-learning/mobile learning, 13, 58, 168–169
question-and-answer sessions, 48, 49, 51
Socratic-type probing, 49
synchronous (real time), 2, 4, 8, 48, 52–53, 60, 74, 77, 80, 121, 130
interactivity, 21, 48, 111, 115, 143, 144
Internet, 2, 3, 5, 8, 27, 53, 54, 65, 72–73, 79, 80, 95, 121, 126, 127, 129, 130, 149, 150, 151

Kirkpatrick model of program evaluation, 101–102

LAAP. *See* Learning Anytime Anywhere Partnerships (LAAP)
learners
adult, 21–22, 25, 26, 28, 110, 141, 153
classroom, 2–3, 6, 7, 25, 27
in a clinical setting, 89–90
generational differences, 9, 47, 55–57. *See also* generation of learners
online. *See* online students
style of. *See* learning style
variable, 39–40, 43
learning
adaptive, 47, 57–58, 120, 169
alternative, 6–7, 16–17
classroom. *See* classroom instruction/classroom teaching; traditional classrooms

178 *Index*

Printed in the United States
By Bookmasters